Newman's

Certified Medical Office Administrative Assistant Study Guide

By Xaiver Newman NRCCS, NRCAHA

Sharnera L. Burgess

TABLE OF CONTENTS

CHAPTER 1: The Medical Assisting Profession

Major Duties Performed by a Medical Administrative Assistant

1. Managing patient registration and communication
2. Scheduling and referral management
3. Managing correspondence
4. Patient or medical records management
5. File system management
6. Office, equipment, and financial management
7. Specific aspects of medication handling
8. Coding, billing, and claims processing
9. Insurance responsibilities
10. Working with managed care plans
11. Credit, billing, and collection
12. Computer operations
13. Banking
14. Accounting and bookkeeping
15. Auditing
16. Complainace Officer

Role of the Medical Administrative Assistant in Educating the Patients

Provide basic information about appointment schedules, billing, insurance services, telephone hours, the physician's office hours, hospital affiliation, reaching the physician after regular office hours, services and facilities including the support services outside of the immediate area to patients who are referred to by other health care facilities.

Employment settings for the Medical Administrative Assistant

Outpatient Facilities.
Inpatient Facilities.
Three-Level Care System.
1. Primary care level
2. Intermediate care level
3. Hospital setting

Professionalism in the Medical Environment

- Support the physician and other staff members in discussions with or about patients.
- First and foremost, always protect the patient's right to confidentiality.
- Accept constructive criticism from the physician, co-workers, or patients without displaying defensive behavior.
- Encourage the patient to ask questions and discuss needs and concerns.
- Resist personal prejudice in patient relations.
- Be aware of the importance of individual presentation; observe the manner and dress of other professionals and strive to present the same professional image.
- Participate in professional organizations that contribute to career enhancement.

- Become highly motivated and apply self-management principles.

Essential Personal Attributes, Basic Technical Skills, and Education

The following are **personal attributes** that are essential in medical assisting:
- Ability to communicate clearly with others
- Common sense
- Diplomacy
- Honesty
- Interest in helping others
- Integrity
- Dependability
- Empathy
- Tolerance
- Sense of humor
- Consideration
- Attentiveness to personal appearance
- Calm manner
- Courtesy

Basic technical skills required of the Medical Administrative Assistant are as follows:
- Mathematics
- Bookkeeping and Banking
- Grammar
- Computers and keyboarding
- Written communication
- Spoken communication and telephone skills
- Medical terminology
- Knowledge of human behavior
- Appointment scheduling/referrals

The **methods of training** to acquire knowledge and skills in medical administrative assisting are as follows:
- On-the-job training.
- Training at a proprietary (private) school.
- Junior college or community college.
- Training from payers (medicare)

Importance of Continuing Education in the Medical Administrative Assisting

1. The practicing medical assistant must keep current with the rapid changes within the profession.
2. Continuing education units (CEUs) are required to maintain certification.

CHAPTER 2:   The HIPAA Compliance

What is HIPAA?

HIPAA, which is also known as the Kennedy-Kassebaum Act, is the acronym for the Health Insurance Portability and Accountability Act of 1996. A federal statute provides for the development of uniform national health information data standards and privacy standards.

The Act includes a section, Title II, entitled Administrative Simplification, requiring:
1.	Improved efficiency in healthcare delivery by standardizing electronic data interchange, and
2.	Protection of confidentiality and security of health data through setting and enforcing standards.

More specifically, HIPAA called upon the Department of Health and Human Services (HHS) to publish new rules that will ensure:
1.	Standardization of electronic patient health, administrative and financial data
2.	Unique health identifiers for individuals, employers, health plans and health care providers; which can be identified as the National Provider Identification number.
3.	Security standards protecting the *confidentiality* and *integrity* of "individually identifiable health information," past, present or future. This information is also known as "Protected Health Information" or PHI.

Who is affected by HIPAA?

Virtually all healthcare organizations – including all health care providers, health plans, public health authorities, healthcare clearinghouses, and self-ensured employers – as well as life insurers, information systems vendors, various service organizations, and universities.

Are There Penalties For Non-Compliance of HIPAA?

HIPAA calls for severe civil and criminal penalties for noncompliance, including:
- o	fines up to $25K for multiple violations of the same standard in a calendar year
- o	fines up to $250K and/or imprisonment up to 10 years for knowing misuse of individually identifiable health information

Generally, what does the HIPAA Privacy Rule require the average provider or health plan to do?

For the average health care provider or health plan, the Privacy Rule requires activities, such as:
- Notifying patients about their privacy rights and how their information can be used.
- Adopting and implementing privacy procedures for its practice, hospital, or plan.
- Training employees so that they understand the privacy procedures.
- Designating an individual to be responsible for seeing that the privacy procedures are adopted and followed.
- Securing patient records containing individually identifiable health information so that they are not readily available to those who do not need them.

The Rules Under HIPAA

HIPAA's **"Administrative Simplification"** provision is composed of four parts, each of which has generated a variety of "rules" promulgated by the Department of Health and Human Services. The four parts of Administrative Simplification are:
1. Standards for Electronic Transactions
2. Unique Identifiers Standards
3. Security Rule
4. Privacy Rule

Privacy Rule

The Privacy Rule is intended to protect the privacy of all individually identifiable health information in the hands of covered entities, regardless of whether the information is or has been in electronic form. The rule establishes the first "set of basic national privacy standards and fair information practices that provides all Americans with a basic level of protection and peace of mind that is essential to their full participation in their care." The Privacy standards:
1. Give patients new rights to access their medical records, restrict access by others, request changes, and to learn how they have been accessed
2. Restrict most disclosures of protected health information to the minimum needed for healthcare treatment and business operations
3. Provide that all patients are formally notified of covered entities' privacy practices,
4. Enable patients to decide if they will authorize disclosure of their protected health information (PHI) for uses other than treatment or healthcare business operations
5. Establish new criminal and civil sanctions for improper use or disclosure of PHI
6. Establish new requirements for access to records by researchers and others
7. Establish business associate agreements with business partners that safeguard their use and disclosure of PHI.
8. Implement a comprehensive compliance program

Confidential Information

All office personnel are responsible for maintaining confidentiality of communication when working with patients and their medical records. **Confidential communication** is privileged communication that may be disclosed only with the patient's permission. Everything you see, hear, or read about patients remains confidential.

Privileged Information

Privileged information is related to the treatment and progress of the patient. The patient must sign an authorization to release this information or selected facts from the medical record. Without this signed authorization, the physician and/or his designee may not release any information about the patient.

Non-privileged Information

Non-privileged information consists of ordinary facts unrelated to treatment of the patient including the patient's name, city of residence, and dates of admission or discharge. This information must be sensitized against unauthorized disclosure under the Privacy section of Health Insurance Portability and Accountability Act (HIPAA). The patient's authorization is needed for the purposes of treatment, payment, or health care operations, unless the record is a specialty hospital (e.g., alcohol treatment) or a special service unit of a general hospital (e.g., psychiatric unit). Professional judgment is required. The information is disclosed on a legitimate need-to-know basis, meaning that the medical data should be revealed to the attending physician because the information may have some effect on the treatment of the patient.

Right to Privacy

All patients have a right to privacy. It is important never to discuss patient information other than with the physician, an insurance company, or individual who has been authorized by the patient.

Exception to the Right to Privacy

Patient records of industrial cases (e.g., workers' compensation), reports of communicable diseases, child abuse, gunshot wounds, and stabbings resulting from criminal actions, and diseases and ailments of newborns and infants. Medical insurance carrier is subject to disclosure to the beneficiary to whom that information pertains. Medical information cannot be accepted by a Medicare insurance carrier from physicians on a confidential basis without the patient's knowledge, either expressed or implied.

Professional Liability

Physicians are legally responsible for their own conduct and any actions of their employees (their designee) performed within the context of their employment. This is referred to as vicarious liability, also known as *respondent superior*, which literally means, "Let the master answer." This does mean that an employee cannot be sued or brought to trial.

Fraud

Fraud is knowing and intentional deception (lying) or misrepresentation that could result in some unauthorized benefit to the deceiver or some other person. It a felony, and if detected, financial or prison penalties can be imposed, depending on the laws of the state. Anyone who has knowledge of fraud or abuse should take the following measures:

1. Notify the provider both personally and with a dated, written memorandum.
2. Document the false statement or representation of the material fact.
3. Send a memorandum to the office manager or employer stating your concern if no change is made.
4. Maintain a written audit trail with dated memoranda.
5. Do not discuss the problem with anyone who is not immediately involved.

Abuse

Abuse means incidents or practices by physicians, not usually considered fraudulent, which are inconsistent with accepted sound medical business or fiscal practices.

Error and Omissions Insurance

Errors and omissions insurance is protection against loss of monies caused by failure through error or unintentional omission on the part of the individual or service submitting the insurance claim.

Embezzlement

Embezzlement means stealing money that has been entrusted in one's care. In many cases of insurance claims embezzlement, the physician is held as the guilty party and has to pay huge sums of money to the insurance carrier when false claims are submitted by an employee.

CHAPTER 3   Medical Practice and Ethics

Definition of Ethics

- **Ethics** are a system of correct conducts from an individual or a group with a single objective.
- **Ethics** is defined as the thoughts, judgments, and actions on issues that have implications of moral right and wrong.
- Ethical systems primarily are concerned with voluntary acts.
- It is assumed that individuals responsible to a code of ethics possess sufficient knowledge and freedom of choice to participate in the system.
- The ethics of a particular profession is the code by which it attempts to regulate the actions of its members and establish general standards.

Medical Ethics for the Medical Administrative Assistant

Code of Ethics provides an ethical foundation for the medical assistant. It provides the latitude necessary to incorporate new information as technological development occurs and serves as a standard of practice for the professional medical assistant. Medical Assistants must be familiar with the five specific guides of conduct in their code. Medical Administrative Assistant's Code of Ethics call for the members to:

- Render service with full respect for the dignity of humanity.
1. Respect confidential information obtained through employment unless legally authorized or required by responsible performance of duty to divulge such information.
2. Uphold the honor and high principles of the profession and accept its disciplines.
3. Seek to continually improve the knowledge and skills of medical assistants for the benefit of patients and professional colleagues.
4. Participate in additional service activities aimed toward improving the health and well being of the community.

Judicial Council of the American Medical Association

- Confidentiality, Advertising, and Communications Media Relations.
1. Information regarding a patient's condition, illness, or disease cannot be released to the press without the consent of the patient or the patient's legal representative.
2. The only situation that does not require the patient's authorization occurs when the information is in the public domain, e.g. births, deaths, accidents, and police cases.
- Fees and Charges.
  4. Fees for medical services must be reasonable, as determined by criteria such as the complexity of the service, the usual and customary fee for the locality, the quality of the services provided, and the experience of the physician.
  5. Fee splitting (paying another health care provider for only the referral of a patient) is always unethical.
  6. Fee should not be charged for routine, simple insurance forms.
  7. Adding interest and finance charges is ethical if the patient is informed in advance.
  8. Billing for certain outside services is done when a laboratory specimen is collected in the physician's office and sent to a clinical laboratory for analysis.
- Physician Records.
  - The progress notes made in a patient's chart and the data gathered are considered the physician's personal property.
  - The information should not be withheld from other physicians, attorneys, or other persons designated by the patient in writing.
  - Record requests accompanied by an appropriate release may not be denied for any reason, including nonpayment of a bill for medical services.
  - On retirement or death of a physician, patients must be notified and their records transferred to the physician of their choice on receipt of written authorization otherwise records should retained by an individual legally permitted to act as a custodian of records.

CHAPTER 4   The Medical Practice and the Law

Medical Practice Acts, their Purpose, and their Relationships to Licensure:
Medical Practice Acts:
1. These are state laws that regulate methods of providing health care to protect the rights and the health of patients. They define the limitation of medical practice, prescribe the penalties for practicing without a valid license, and specify the conditions warranting the revocation of a physician's license.

Common Reasons for the Revocation of a Medical license:
- Drug addiction or substance abuse.
- Felony conviction.
- Crime involving moral turpitude.
- Prescribing drugs without examining the patient or performing a good-faith examination of the patient.
- Insurance claim fraud.
- Gross negligence in the care of patients.

Law of Contracts Governing the Medical Practice:
Establishing a Physician-Patient Relationship.
1. Patient care is established by mutual agreement between the physician and the patient.
2. This agreement is a contract, whether it is **expressed**[1] or **implied**.[2]
3. **Contractual agreement** result from the following events: physicians make their services available, patients accept those services by requesting treatment, and physicians begin to treat patients.

Patient Expectations from the Medical Practice
Careful and consistent patient education and the establishment of an open communications system are important.

Procedural Steps to be Observed in Terminating a Contract with the Patient
- Patient refusal to follow advice or cooperate in the agreed treatment program or failure to keep appointment continually is among the causes of the Physician's termination of relationship with the patient.
- The physician-patient relationship must be terminated when the physician retires, relocates, or discontinues practice for any reason.

---

[1] An *expressed contract* is a formal contract, usually in distinct written or oral language.
[2] Most patient care contracts are *implied*; they are not produced by or documented in an explicit agreement between the physician and the patient.

- If the physician decides to terminate the relationship with the patient, the following are the procedural steps that may be observed:
  - Gather necessary materials.
  - Follow guidelines in office policy and procedures manual to write letter indicating the physician's decision to withdraw from the relationship.
  - The letter should advise the patient of the following: the physician's care is being discontinued and the physician will turn over the patient's records to the patient or to another physician.
  - Send the letter by certified mail and request a return receipt.
  - Place a photocopy of the letter in the patient's file.
  - When the receipt is returned, attached it to the photocopy of the letter in the patient's file.
- Patients may also choose to terminate care by the physician.
- The patient charge **abandonment** unless the physician does the following:
  1. Provides adequate notification of the intention to terminate care.
  2. Remains available to the patient during the notification period.
  3. Provides competent substitute care is necessary.
  4. Cooperate with the new physician by supplying the information necessary to provide appropriate care.

Concept on Standards of Care

In legal sense, the **standard of care** is determined by the care that would be provided by an average practitioner under the same or similar conditions. In all cases, physicians are expected to fulfill the following obligations:
- Apply their best judgment in diagnosis and treatment.
- Refer a patient to a specialist or request consultation when necessary.
- Advise patients of their physical condition, limitations, or need for continued care.

Professional Liability in the Medical Practice

- State laws generally involve two types of actions and responsibilities: criminal and civil.
- **Criminal law** deals with actions that are punishable as offenses against the state.
- **Civil law** involves the actions of individuals against individuals and is covered by the segment of the law known as *tort*.
- Professional liability claims must have the following two components to be valid:
  o The physician fails in his or her duty to a patient as required by the medical practice acts.
  o The failure in duty results in a discernable injury to the patient.
- The common term for professional liability is *malpractice*, a word that medical professionals dislike because of its negative connotation.
- The use of the word *malpractice* should always be avoided when performing professional duties; use the term *medical professional liability* instead.
- The common reasons for lawsuits are as follows: negligence, lack of informed consent, abandonment, and missed diagnosis.
- Negligence in the performance of duty constitutes malpractice in any profession and it is a result of an action or an omission.
- Physicians are negligent if they perform a service that is not in accordance with the expected standards of care or fail to perform a service necessary for the well-being of a patient.

Criteria of Negligence

A physician's liability (responsibility) is determined to exist if the following exists:

- *Duty* - Mutual agreement (usually implied) establishes a contract for medical care between the physician and the patient. Once a physician accepts the responsibility for a patient's care, the physician has a duty to provide medical services according to the standards of care.
- *Derelict* - The derelict physician fails in the performance of duty to the patient by either falling short of the expected standards of care or abandoning the patient.
- *Direct cause* - The principle of direct cause means that an explicit act or omission by the physician is directly linked to the injury suffered by the patient. The plaintiff must prove that the physician's actions or lack of action, and no other possible cause, resulted in an injury.
- *Damages* - These are the result of actions by a physician that could have been predicted or anticipated.

ABCD's of Negligence

    A: Acceptance of a person as a patient
    B: Breach of the physician's duty of skill or care
    C: Casual connection between the breach by the physician and the damage to the patient.
    D: Damage of foreseeable nature.

Statue of Limitations

Each state determines a statue of limitations, the time during which civil lawsuit may be filed. Medical Administrative Assistant's Roles in preventing civil suits.

i. All patient information obtained from or about the patient must only be exchanged with staff members in private.
ii. When calling in prescription, medical assistants should always take care that they are not in an area where other patients can listen to or observe information regarding other patients and their prescription.
iii. The patient should always be protected from unnecessary or inappropriate physical exposure.
iv. The medical assistant should never discuss a particular patient or case outside the office, even when the patient's name is withheld.
v. An exception is made for professional discussions, such as referral of a patient to another office or use of the patient's case (but not the name or facts that may identify the patient) in class.
vi. Charts and written documents regarding a patient should be kept out of view of other patient and visitors to the office.

Good Samaritan Acts

Good Samaritan Acts encourage voluntary help by protecting physician from legal liability under civil law. These statutes generally make the physician immune from any lawsuit arising out of emergency care, if the help is given with reasonable care under the circumstances and in good faith. It does not protect the physician in professional setting such as medical offices, clinics, and hospitals.

CHAPTER 5   The Role of the Medical Administrative Assistant as a Receptionist

Interpersonal Skills and Human Behavior Required of a Medical Administrative Assistant
Patient who visit the healthcare facility may not be at their best, and the way in which the medical assistant reacts and interacts with them can make an incredible difference in their perception of the office, the physician, and the medical staff.

First Impressions include attitude and compassion, and the all-important smile.

Communication Paths both Verbal and Non-verbal
Verbal communication depends on words and sounds.
- The *pitch* of the voice is a part of verbal communication.
- The medical assistant should speak clearly and enunciate words properly.
- Eye contact and the tone of the voice are both critical and vital in verbal communication.
- There is no place for sarcasm or caustic remarks in verbal communication.

Nonverbal communications are messages conveyed without the use of words. They are transmitted by body language, gestures, and mannerisms that may or may not be in agreement with the words a person speaks. It involves eye contact, facial expression, hand gestures, grooming, and dress, and space, tone of voice, posture, and touch.

Our need for personal space is demonstrated by how patients in the reception area will choose a seat. The acceptable distance for personal space when communicating with a patient ranges from 1.5 to 4 feet.

Process of Communications must be clear and concise, and the message we intend to send must match what the receiver understands.

Elements in the communication process.
- When two people interact, both people act as a sender and as receiver.
- The sender is the person who sends a message through a variety of different channels.
- Channels can be spoken words, written messages, and body languages.
- The sender encodes the message, which simply means that he or she chooses a specific way of expression using words and other channels.
- The receiver decodes the message according to his or her understanding of what is being communicated.

Noise is anything that interferes with the message being sent which can be external, internal, and physiological.

Listening - Look at the speaker and pay attention. Be diligent in not only hearing the words being spoken, but also listening to them and what the patient is attempting to communicate.

Active listening is the skill whereby paraphrasing and clarifying what the speaker has said takes place.

Paraphrasing is listening to what the sender is communicating, analyzing the words, and then restating them to confirm that the receiver has understood the message as the sender intended it.

Rules that Must be Observed by the Medical Administrative Assistant in Advising Patient

The medical assistant must be extremely careful when giving advice to a patient in order to avoid legal accusations of practicing medicine without a license. Strict laws in most states prohibit anyone other than a license physician from giving medical advice. Patients must come to their own decisions about treatments and options that they have when faced with a medical decision. The medical assistant is often looked on not only as an authority figure, but also as an extension of the physician. Patients may mistakenly think that the medical assistant reflects the same opinion as the physician.

Responsibilities of the Medical Administrative Assistant as a Receptionist

Greeting Visitors.

1. Patient, who is the most important visitors in your office, must be greeted warmly.
2. Your role is linked to the appointment system.
3. You are the first person to greet patients as they arrive and therefore make the first impression.
4. The tone of your greeting, as well as appearance will set the tone of the visit.

Elements in creating a positive first impression.

- *Attitude* – Establish the initial impression of the office and of its personnel that are based on general appearance, etiquette, and the appearance of the work environment.
- *Appearance* – Includes appropriate dress, tasteful make-up and accessories, and proper hygiene.
- *Etiquette* – The Medical Assistant should be courteous in welcoming people and greet person by name.

Dealing with patients waiting for services.

- Never ignore patients in the reception area.

Dealing with other waiting in the reception area.

1. *Children* - Plan for their presence, that is furnishings and recreational materials should be appropriate and safe for them.
2. *Relatives or Friends of the Patient* - Let them know the approximate time the patient's visit will be completed. Be careful not answer questions regarding the patient's condition or treatment.

Important Factors to be considered in Managing the Reception Area

The reception area should be pleasant, well-lighted area in which patients and visitors can wait comfortably. Desks should be kept neatly arranged. After arriving at the office each morning, check the reception area to see that everything is neat and clean, with all magazines arranged attractively. Current magazine should be available in an area they can be replaced easily and appropriate for clientele.

The seating should be attractively arranged, with a variety of seating options. Artwork in the reception area reflects the taste of the physician-owner but should be relatively conservative in color and design. Check the reception area frequently to see whether patients are still waiting and straighten the room when you have a free moment.

Patient Registration

Before the patient arrives, the assistant checks the name on the appointment sheet and watches for the patient's arrival. Ask established patients whether there are any changes in their personal information such as new address, telephone number, place of employment, and insurance plan. Any patient arriving for a first visit requires certain introductory procedures.

Considerations that Must be Given to the Patient

Do what you can to ensure the patient sees the physician at the appointed time, or very close to it. Consideration for the patient's time is extremely important. If the patient is already in the reception area and the wait becomes excessive, (more than 20 minutes) you should explain the delay to the patient. Consideration for elderly and disabled patients is as follows:

- Reserve time for the first appointment after lunch.
- Speak clearly and slowly.
- Provide assistance in filing out patient information and patient registration forms in a well-lit area.
- Be knowledgeable about which insurance plans the physician accepts.
- Provide surgical instructions in large and bold type.
- Provide information sheets on special subjects related to geriatric patients.
- Provide refrigerator magnets that include the physician's name and telephone number.
- Maintain a warm temperature in the examination rooms.
- Add the name and telephone of the patients nearest relative, close friend, attorney, or clergy to the patient's chart.
- Insure that HIPAA compliance forms are filled-up or the release of information is executed.

Patient's Complaints

Learn to listen and project a feeling of empathy as well as be aware that no complaint, no matter how small or big, is to be ignored.

How to Deal with Upset Patient and Excessive Talkers

Remain calm and sure of yourself. Try to understand why the patient is upset (empathy) and do not raise your voice or become agitated. Have a prearranged signal to alert the physician that the next patient has arrived, which will allow the physician to exit gracefully.

Discrimination in the Office

Discrimination. – is defined as "unfair treatment of a person because of race, sex, religious affiliation, or disability." In handling discrimination, you must learn how to recognize discriminating behavior and refuse to accept it.

Office Emergencies

- Office Emergencies.
  - Maintain a flexible attitude so that you can adjust on a moment's notice.
  - React calmly in a situation that demands immediate attention.

CHAPTER 6   Telephone Skills

Importance of Telephone Communication

It is a vital part of the medical practice. The Medical Administrative Assistant has a responsibility to patients and physicians to develop effective techniques of oral communication. It is the lifeline of a medical practice as well as powerful public relations tool. Medical assistants must remember that the voice on the other end of the line is that of the patient, and telephone calls can never be considered an interruption of the workday.

Incoming Calls

Incoming calls make up approximately 80% of the daily telephone activity in an office or agency. Up to 50% of this activity involves patients or potential patients. Most incoming calls are from these sources:

1. Established patients calling for appointments or to ask questions.
2. Individuals reporting emergencies.
3. Other physicians who are making referrals.
4. Laboratories reporting vital information regarding a patient.
5. New Patients making a first contact with the physician's office.

How to Use the Telephone Effectively

Active Listening: The same importance, as in face-to-face conversation, should be given to active listening when answering telephone. It provides vital information about the nature of the call-whether the caller is distressed and agitated or has a concern that needs to be addressed immediately.

Developing a Pleasing Telephone Voice.
Individuals who call a physician's office should hear a pleasant, friendly voice when they greeted. It is a common sales technique to be sure that the caller "hears a smile." Be sure to enunciate words clearly, pronouncing then separately and distinctly. Diction, pitch, and clarity are important. Avoid speaking in a monotone; instead, use inflection, or a change in the pitch and volume of your voice when speaking. Always use friendly and warm tone of voice and project confidence when speaking with patients. Be courteous and tactful and choose words carefully. Every caller should be made to feel that the

medical assistant has time to attend to his or her wishes. A small mirror, placed near the telephone, will serve as a reminder to smile. Be alert and interested in the person who is calling.

Always give full attention to the caller and do not allow distractions from the conversation. Build a pleasant, friendly image for the office. Talk naturally and avoid repetition of mechanical words and phrases, such as "uh huh" and "you know" and "like." Avoid the use of professional jargon, such as referring to "Otis Media" when the patient is reporting an earache. Using correct grammar adds to the caller's favorable impression.

Talk directly into the mouthpiece. Never answer the telephone when eating, drinking, or chewing gum. Use a normal tone of voice speaking neither too loud nor too soft and at a moderate or normal rate.

Never release information about a patient's health or other protected information or offer medical advice. The physician should answer all medical questions.

Telephone's General Courtesy Techniques
1.   Answer promptly, preferably on the first or second ring.
2.   Hold the instrument properly.
3.   Identify the office and yourself.
4.   Use the hold button properly.

Telephone Etiquette
Remember that the first 15 seconds of a phone call are crucial. Telephone skills can "make or break" the practice. Some good advice is as follows:
- Use your natural voice
- Sit up straight
- Answer calls with a smile
- Address your patients appropriately
- Notice the response of your callers
- Listen actively
- Obtain needed information

When interrupting a call to answer another call, the suggested steps to be observed are as follows:
- Excuse yourself from the person on the line and explain that you have another call coming in and that you will be right back.
- Answer the second call, and put the second caller on hold as previously suggested.
- Return to the first caller, thank him or her for waiting, and mention that the other line is on hold.

When answering a call, and you are unable to complete the conversation.
- Answer promptly
- Hold the instrument properly
- Identify the office and yourself
- Allow the caller to identify himself or herself

- Restate the caller's name
- Ask the caller if he or she can hold for a moment
- Wait for the caller's reply
- Thank the caller and depress the hold button
- When you return to the call, thank the caller again and continue with the conversation

Handling Calls.
- Be prepared
- Get the information you need
- Control the call
- Log the call

Telephone Techniques in Handling Troublesome Callers

<u>Angry Caller:</u> Remain calm and determine the issue. Assure the caller that you are interested in helping.

<u>Repeat Caller:</u> Maybe eliminated by providing patients with printed instructions that has been prepared for routine situations in your office. If the caller persists, you may suggest scheduling an appointment to discuss the concerns with the doctor.

<u>Appointment Juggler:</u> Remind patients the importance of keeping the appointment and let them know that it helps to have more notice when they cannot keep an appointment since another patient could be scheduled.

<u>Caller Seeking Aid beyond Your Duties:</u> should be declined tactfully and direct the call to the appropriate person.

<u>Caller Requesting Confidential Information.</u> All communications in a healthcare facility are confidential. Tell the caller that the patient's written consent is necessary to release the information A call from an institution stating that they admitted your patient and need information from the patient's record, should be appropriately handled as follows:
1. Request some identifying data on the patient, such as date of birth or Social Security Number
2. Request the caller's name and telephone number, stating that you will call back immediately after pulling the patient's chart for the physician. By returning the call, you can verify the institution and person to whom you are speaking.

<u>The Unidentified Caller:</u> If you receive calls from individuals who refuse to identify themselves or who misrepresent their identity or the nature of their business, be guided by your office policy, which will direct you on how to deal with calls of this type.

Outgoing Calls

1. <u>Telephone Etiquette</u> - Calls should be designed to save time and respect the other person's needs.
2. <u>Planning Your Calls</u> - Locate the correct telephone number. Compile the information needed during the call. Keep a notepad and writing instruments nearby.
3. <u>Dialing Errors</u> - Apologize to the person you disturbed.
4. <u>Use of Directories</u> - Directories should be readily available to all personnel who place outgoing calls. The office should acquire as many directories as necessary to avoid frequently moving them from one site to another.

CHAPTER 7   Appointment Scheduling

Types of Appointment Scheduling Systems

1. Open Office Hours.
   - It is the least structured and least commonly used method of scheduling patients and an inefficient method of time management. Patients are advised that the office is open during a certain block of time, such as from noon to 4:00 PM, and they may come in anytime between those hours.
   - Scheduled Appointments.
   4. Patients call the office to schedule an appointment. It is the most efficient scheduling system.
   a. Flex Hours.
      2. The practice offers extended or flexible office hours. This practice gives the patient numerous options which is best suited to group practices or partnerships consisting of four or more physicians because more physicians are available for time rotation.

Formula for Effective Appointment

1. *The doctor*-who arrives on time and sees patients in a timely manner.
2. *The patient*-who schedules in advance as much as possible, and who is on time for appointments or who calls in advance when an appointment cannot be kept.
3. *The Medical Administrative Assistant*-who schedules the patient to meet with the doctor (the appointment) and looks at the time, length, and necessity of appointment to make these arrangements.

Considerations to be Observed in Scheduling

The method of scheduling appointments should be individualized for the specialty or practice. The specifics of the area served such as agricultural, industrial, or retirement community. Keep in mind the following considerations: *patient needs, work or school schedules, childcare needs, special needs, and physician's habits and preferences.*

Guidelines for Scheduling Office Appointments

Know the patients, in advance if possible, who you will be seeing each day and for what reasons you will be seeing them.

1. Necessary Information From the Patient In Making Advance Appointments: *patient's full name, daytime telephone number, reason for the visit, referral source, and insurance/payment information for new patients.*
2. Necessary Information for the Patient.
   a. Patient has the correct information.
   b. State the appointment day, date, and time as you note the patient's name in the appointment book or computer listing, and state them again before you complete the call.
3. Follow-Up Appointments
   a. Try to schedule the next appointment while the patient is still in the office.
4. Scheduling Appointments by Telephone.
   a. After the date and time have been agreed on, you may send the patient a written appointment card and, for new patients, a patient information brochure in a sealed envelop to comply with HIPAA requirements.
5. New Patient Appointment Guidelines.
   a. New patient need to feel comfortable with the office.
   b. Get their full names, daytime phone numbers, and reason for the visit.
   c. Get the referral source and insurance information.
   d. Explain any office policies that the new patient should know before coming to your office.
   e. Tell them how to get to the office (give specific directions and if there is time, mail an office map).
   f. Try to give them some idea of how long their visit may take. Many practices devote at least 30 to 45 minutes for the first visit.

Appointment Management Techniques

1. __Time-Specified__ - Each patient is given an appointment for a definite time.
2. __Wave__ - It provides flexibility and is designed to self-adjust to the unpredictable variances caused by patients. It is based on the average time spent with each patient on a routine visit.
3. __Modified Wave -__ This is similar to the wave system wherein an hour is the base block of time. The modification involves pre-spacing the arrival time of the patients planned for a given hour.
4. __Double Booking__ - Double booking is a form of wave scheduling and occurs when two patients, both requiring the physician's attention for the total appointment slot are scheduled for the same time.
5. __Grouping Procedures__ - Book similar examinations or procedures within specific blocks of time. It may be in response to an anticipated special situation or may be routine occurrence

Scheduling by Exception

This refers to unplanned situations that require an immediate appointment. These situations can include: *emergency patients, acute-need patients, referrals, and for special situations.*

Scheduling Diagnostic Studies (Outpatient)

1. **Appointment Scheduling** -The Medical assistant is usually responsible for scheduling these studies because of the medical terminology that may be involved.
2. **Scheduling Information** - You will need to supply certain information that you have gathered before placing the call, including the following: name, age, or date of birth, insurance carrier, and suspected diagnosis or reason for study.
3. **Patient Instructions** - The Medical Assistant may provide the patient with pre-printed forms for special instructions which you may review with the patient.

Disruption in the Appointment System

Should be kept to a minimum and the patient's needs and comfort should be foremost in your mind. Common causes of scheduling disruptions are as follows: patient failure to keep appointments, patients cancellations, delayed arrival of the physician, and physician absence because of an emergency

Steps to be Performed When Patient Failed to Keep Appointment

✓ The cancellation must be noted in the appointment book.
✓ A single line should be drawn through the name and the reason for the cancellation noted.
✓ The single line indicates the appointment was not kept, and the name can still be read and verified.
✓ Note N/S (for no-show) or F/S (failed to show) for the patient who does not arrive.
✓ "C" or "canc" should be noted after the name of an individual who cancels an appointment.
✓ Note the date of the new appointment if one is made or note "w/c" for with call, if the patient states he or she will reschedule at another time.

Steps to be Performed When Patient Failed to Keep Appointment Without Notification

✓ Handling Techniques.
   3. If you contact the patient or the patient calls the office, you should be courteous and understanding and schedule another appointment.
   4. If the situation occurs repeatedly, you will have to explain diplomatically the problems that result.
   5. When repeated failure to keep appointments interferes with proper care of a patient, the physician may choose to dismiss him or her.
- Recording - Should be recorded in the appointment book and in the patient's chart.

Steps to be Performed When Patient Failed to Keep Appointment
With Notification
1. Rescheduling - Attempt to reschedule it during the same telephone call.
2. Notations - Cancellations should be noted in the appointment book and the patient's chart along with the date of the rescheduled appointment.
i. Use of Time - Offer the appointment time to another patient. If it is a late cancellation, the time may be used to accomplish other duties.

Steps to be observed when the Physician is delayed in arriving to the office for a reasonable period.
Reasons and Staff Notification.
- Remind the physician occasionally of the importance of staff notification.

Notifying Patients.
- Explain the situation to the patients who have already arrived.
- Attempt to reach patients by telephone in the order that they are scheduled to arrive at the office.
- Patients in transit to the office will have to receive an explanation of the situation when they arrive.
- The rest of the patients can be notified at home or work before leaving for the appointment.
- Each patient should be offered the option of either waiting for the physician to arrive or rescheduling the appointment.

Importance of Effective Appointment Management
Patients' most frequent complaint is the time spent in the office reception area. If the delay is unusual, keep the patients informed about the reason for the delay and the anticipated time involved. If delays are common, reevaluate the system and observe the staff members' effects on the efficiency of the system.

Acceptable Wait. Surveys and evaluation of patient questionnaires both show that the maximum acceptable wait in an office before seeing the physician is 20 minutes.

CHAPTER 8   Correspondence and Mail Management

Importance of Written Communication
Written communication is the unspoken exchange of ideas between individuals, who in many instances have never met one another. The manner in which you handle communication responsibilities will affect the efficiency of the office.

<u>**Advantageous Features of Word Processing**</u>
- Personalization of multiple letters.
- Rapid drafting or revision of lengthy documents.
- Capacity for adding, deleting, and moving words, phrases, sentences, and paragraphs without retyping the entire page or document.
- Automatic alignment of figures, tables, and graphs for statistical reports.
- Spell check.
- Thesaurus.
- Change of fonts.

<u>**Sorting Mail**</u>
If the mail has been properly sorted and stacked, the items you can expect to see, from top to bottom, will be:
- Telegrams; faxes; express, certified, registered, and priority mail
- E-mail, personal letters, business correspondence from other professionals
- Payments from patients, insurance forms, invoices, letters regarding accounts
- Medical reports, laboratory and x-ray reports
- Professional materials, meeting announcements, medical bulletins
- Medical journals, journal reprints
- Magazines, newspaper
- Pharmaceutical literature or samples
- Advertisements

<u>**Outgoing Correspondence, Punctuation, Transcription, Editing and Proofreading, Letter Styles, and Parts of the Letter**</u>
1. Spelling.
   - Correct spelling is vital to the impression transmitted by written communication.
   - Use the appropriate dictionary for correct spelling or spell check when using word processor.
   - Even if you use spell check, you must proofread your correspondence.
2. Punctuation.
   1. Standard methods of punctuation should be used throughout all correspondence.
3. Transcription.
   - One must have taken courses in medical terminology and used dictation equipment, and be fully familiar with medical procedures handled within the practice.
   - The quality of transcription may be influenced by the quality of dictation, but experience usually compensates for handling dictation.
   o Editing and Proofreading.
      ▪ For important communication or communication that is still in the developmental stage, make a rough draft which may be typed on inexpensive papers.
      ▪ Comments and changes at this stage are referred to as editing.
      ▪ Once the draft is acceptable, the material can be prepared in final form.

1. Letter Styles.
   - Blocked
   - Semi-Blocked
   - Full-Blocked

Correspondence Generated by the Medical Administrative Assistant

Most outgoing office communication is the responsibility of the medical assistant. The skill and timeliness with which this communication is handled will reflect on the assistant and ultimately on the physician. Each letter that is release from a medical office reveals subtle information about the intelligence, ability, and efficiency of the writer.

Some of the Medical Administrative Assistant's correspondence responsibilities include:
3. Responses to patient inquiries on administrative procedures.
4. Exchanges with suppliers and business associates.
5. Account collections.
6. Exchanges with insurance companies.
7. Notification to patients of surgery or hospital arrangements.
8. Letters of solicitation.

Special Mail Services

Certified Mail.
1. It provides a record of delivery that is retained at the addressee's post office for 2 years.
2. A return receipt, signed by the addressee or addressee's agent, can be acquired and returned to the sender to verify that the item was received.

Express Mail.
3. It is fast, intercity delivery system geared to the special needs of business and industry.
4. It offers reliable transfer of time-sensitive documents and products.

Insured Mail.
5. Third-class and fourth-class mail may be insured against loss and damage up to $400.

Mailgrams.
6. This is a special service offered jointly by the U.S. Postal Service and Western Union.
7. Messages charged at 100-word units may be dictated by telephone to Western Union, which transmit them to the destination city for next-day delivery by the postal service.

Priority Mail.
8. It is a special service for first-class mail that weighs more than 11 ounces but not more than 70 pounds.
9. It is fastest way to get heavier mail to its destination, with a 2- or 3-day delivery assured.

Registered Mail.
10. First class and priority mail may be registered if the contents are valuable.
11. The value of the item is declared by the sender.

12. The fee for this service is based on the declared value of the item, and the sender is given a receipt that must be retained until the item is received by the addresses.

Electronic Mail or Email.
2. A system for exchanging written messages (and increasingly, voice and video messages) through a network.
3. It is fast and inexpensive way to communicate with other people.
4. It offers reliable transfer of time-sensitive documents.
5. It can be transmitted to multiple people in various locations at the same time.
6. Retain and save copies for documentation.

CHAPTER 9   Patients and Medical Records Management

Importance of Records Management
Records management is the development and maintenance of a systematic method of receiving, processing, and gathering paper for storage. The main purpose of keeping accurate and complete medical records is to assist in giving the best possible care and treatment to the patient.

Purpose of Records Management
- Single Location of Data.
- Continuum of Information.
- Comprehensive Record of Data From Various Sources.
- Rapid Retrieval of Information
- Legal Protection of the Patient Confidentiality.
- Protecting Patient's Identities.
- Release of Records.
- Protection of the Physician.
- Permanent Protection.
- Statistical Information.

Legal Consideration Regarding Entries in the Medical Record
The entries in a medical record are unalterable. Entries to be avoided - A thoughtless comment, humorous or sarcastic remarks should never be written in a patient's record.

Medical Record as a Legal "Safe"
It is vital that the record be an accurate, complete document so that the physician can:
1. Protect him or her in court by being able to prove that he or she gave adequate treatment, that is, "the standard of care."
2. Support insurance company billings with the correct coding justification.
3. Use the information recorded to complete the reports required by law in the case of child abuse, communicable disease, and criminal action such as gunshot wounds or stabbings.

Organization of the Medical Record
Physician's notes
1. The physician's notes begin with the information history and initial evaluation.
2. Subsequent visits are noted on sheets called *progress notes*.
3. The notes are stamped with the date of each visit.

4. Most physician prefer that progress notes, the first section encountered when the chart cover is opened, be maintained in reverse chronological order, with the sheet describing the most recent visit on top and the oldest entry on the bottom.

Diagnostic and hospital records
- When monitoring the patient's condition, the physician frequently refers to this section. Progress usually is stored in reverse chronological order, with the most recently dated report on top.
- Some common subsections are as follows: *progress notes, consultation, laboratory, x-ray, operative reports, correspondence, prescription and medication as well as correspondence which contains letters and narrative reports from physicians or facilities that previously have provided care for the patient, insurance forms, and copies of insurance forms prepared by the Medical Administrative Assistant.*

Styles of Progress Notes
1. *Narrative* - It is the oldest method. After the administrative assistant writes in the date, chief complaint, and vital signs, the physician notes, what was wrong with the patient, his or her examination findings, and what treatment he or she is using.
2. *SOAP-* It is used with a problem-oriented medical record and means Subjective, Objective, Assessment, and Plan. Subjective is what the patient says is wrong. Objective is what is seen in the examination of the patient, including vital signs and tests. Assessment is the physician's impression of what is wrong with the patient. Plan is what is going to be done for the patient, that is, medication, special tests, referrals, return in 10 days, and so on.

Deletions and Corrections of Medical Records
Only the physician should decide what specific material might be deleted from an office medical record. Medical administrative assistants should never take it upon themselves to make such a decision, even if an exact duplicate of a report already is in the record. It is recommended by most medical associations that documentation removed from patient charts either be microfilmed or retained in a permanent storage area.

Typical Material Deleted.
1. Duplicates of diagnostic studies.
2. Hospital studies over 3 years old (the hospital will have the originals if needed) that show normal findings; retain any report of abnormal findings.
3. Insurance forms over 7 years old.
4. Individual progress notes or pages of notes should never be deleted from a medical record.

Protecting Confidentiality
Extreme care must be taken to make sure that material removed from the patient's chart is disposed of properly. No one should be able to discern the patient's name or connect the name with a report when it is discarded. Shredding the report may be a good option.

Corrections, Maintenance of Medical Records, and Period of Records Retention

- Correction Technique.
  1. Step 1: Strike a single line through the error.
  2. Step 2: Date and initial the strikeout.
  3. Step 3: If the problem is incorrect data, enter the corrected information directly below the strikeout.
  4. Step 4: If the entry is made in the chart, follow step 1 and note, "Recorded in chart by error. Information transferred to chart of John C. Adams." Date and sign the strikeout and explanation.
  5. Step 4 is vital for legal purposes, because it can be verified. It is not considered a breach of confidentiality.
- Maintenance of Medical Records.
  1. It is the responsibility of the Medical Administrative Assistant to see that the medical records must be constantly and methodically kept current.
  2. You should continually attempt to maintain and improve medical records management.
- Transfer and Retention of Medical Records.
  - Each office must establish a policy when a record should be considered inactive and transferred to storage.
  - In most situations this will depend on: age of the chart (date since last visit), type of practice, space available in the "active" filing cabinets.
  - Many offices find that 2 to 3 years since the last visit is an appropriate time span for considering a record for storage.
  - Closed charts should be transferred within 6 months which include; patients who have died, moved away and did not request their chart, and terminated their relationship with the physician.
- Period of Records Retention.
  - When care involves a minor, the record should always be kept at least until the patient is 21 years old, and thereafter until the local statue of limitations runs outs.
  - Closure of a case, as in a specialist's care, may warrant destroying a chart after a given time period.
  - Most agree that the chart should be retained for at least 10 years.
  - After the uncomplicated death of a patient, some professionals suggest that the chart be retained through the statue of limitations and then destroyed.
  - In the event of a physician's retirement, the charts of deceased patients may be destroyed after a selected time period following the death and following appropriate notification of the next of kin.
  - The records of living patients may be transferred to the physician continuing the practice or to a physician of the patient's choice on receipt of written authorization.
  - On the death of a physician, the patient's records are put under the care of a custodian of records, who often is the physician's spouse or a former employee who is willing to perform the duties involved.
- General Advice.
  1. The only safe option for records retention is to retain them forever that is, it should not be destroyed.

Medical Record Protection

1. Records Temporarily Out of File.
   a. You must protect and pay particular attention to medical records that are out of the office because they were subpoenaed.
   b. If you must send a record out, be certain to photocopy at least the doctor's notes, since they can never be replaced.
   c. Keep a record of charts that must be sent out, the date they are sent, and to whom they are sent.
   d. If the chart has not returned within 10 days, contact the subpoena service and ask them to locate the record and notify you regarding when it will be returned. This encounter should be properly documented by recording the name of the contact person, the date and time as well as the response.
2. After-Office Hours.
   1. At the end of each day all possible records should be returned to the filing cabinet for security purposes.
   2. The filing cabinets should be closed and, if possible, locked.
3. Records Removed by Physician.
   - All malpractice carriers advise physicians to never remove medical records from the office.
4. Destruction of Medical Records.
   - Each state has a statue of limitations regarding how long to keep medical records.
   - You may destroy records, as stated earlier, only after checking with the physician's malpractice carrier and attorney.

CHAPTER 10   Filing

Filing Systems and Procedures
1. Correct filing is necessary for every medical office.
2. It is essential in every office that the file clerk, which is one of the major team players, be interested in keeping the office organized and on schedule.

Four Basic Filing Systems
1. Alphabetical by name.
   a. Is the easiest and most commonly used system for organizing patients' records.
   b. Labeled folders are arranged in the same sequence as the letters of the alphabet.
2. Numerical.
   a. Materials are categorized first by number and second by an alphabetical cross-reference.
   b. Each new patient is assigned a number in sequence; this may be the account number assigned by the computer billing system.
   c. A cross-reference is established after the number has been assigned.
   d. Either an index card or ledger card is arranged alphabetically and followed by the previously assigned numerical code.
   e. There are two types of numerical filing systems, namely: **consecutive system** and **terminal digit system**.
   f. In the **consecutive system**, individuals are assigned numbers consecutively as patients come to the practice.

g. In the **terminal digit system**, patients are given consecutive numbers but the digits are separated into groups of two or three and are read in groups from right to left.
  i. Records are filed backward in groups as follows:
     02 88 00
     00 70 01
     04 44 11
     01 65 20
     89 33 22
     90 33 22
  1. The advantages of the numerical system are its capacity for expansion without rearrangement of the cabinets (as in alphabetical filing) and clear identification of individuals with similar or identical names.
3. Geographical.
  a. Filing according to the patient's place of residence is a technique normally used in major clinics or medical centers and must be cross-referenced by an alphabetical system.
  b. This system may be used in facilities wishing to gather statistical data or trying to locate a disease process within a geographical area.
4. Subject.
  a. Subject filing may be used for patient records as a cross-index if the physician is interested in gathering statistics on various disease processes.
  b. You will use subject filing in the business aspect of the practice for keeping information and correspondence in appropriate categories.
  c. Folders are prepared and labeled to store information on subjects such as equipment maintenance contracts, office policies, office procedures, worker's compensation injury reports, etc.

Steps in Filing
1. Examination.
2. Indexing.
3. Coding.
4. Sorting.
5. Storing.

Rules of Indexing
1. Indexing is based on dividing a name into units.
2. Units are numbered beginning with 1.
3. Three units are usually sufficient for the use in the average medical practice.
4. A detailed description of the rules of indexing is presented as follows:

- *Person's names are indexed with the last name as Unit 1, the given (first) name as Unit 2, and the middle name or initial as Unit 3. For example, John C. Jones is indexed as:*

  Unit 1   **Unit 2**   **Unit 3**
  Jones   John   C.

- *Once in units, the names are read from left to right, compared, and then placed in alphabetical order according to the first letter that differs. Thus, Jones, Jane A. will be filed before Jones, John C. because the "a" in Jane is the first letter that differs alphabetically from the "o" in John.*

- *Initials used in place of a first name are considered a unit and placed before a spelled-out name. Thomas Jones, J. or Jones, J. Charles is placed before Jones, John C.*

- *Any hyphenated name is considered a single unit; the hyphen is disregarded. Thus Clayton-Moore, Sylvia is indexed as:*

  Unit 1   **Unit 2**
  Claytonmoore   Sylvia

- *Apostrophes are disregarded in indexing. Thus Morton's Pharmacy is read as Mortons Pharmacy.*

- *Names with foreign prepositions or articles are filed as one unit, and the space between the preposition or article and the name is ignored. Thus Claude de Mason is read and indexed as:*

  Unit 1   **Unit 2**
  Demason   Claude

- *Abbreviated portions of names are read and indexed as of written in full. Thus Mary St. John is indexed as:*

  Unit 1   **Unit 2**   **Unit 3**
  Saint   John   Mary

- *The prefixes Mac and Mc may be filed in one of two ways: (1) You may use individual dividers to establish a separate section for all Mc's and another for all Mac's. These would become a subsystem within the files in which the name following the prefix becomes the first indexing unit. Following the Mac divider, the names MacDonald, MacAndrew, MacHenry in proper order would be indexed as:*

  Unit 1   **Unit 2**   **Unit 3**
  Andrew   Elizabeth   D.
  Donald   Joseph
  Henry   Sharon   L.

  Mc would be the next divider and include names organized in the same way as those under Mac. The dividers would then resume the normal alphabetical order. (2) You may disregard the prefix and threat it the same as indicated in Rule 4. Thus MacDonald, MacHenry, and MacAndrew would be read, indexed, and filed as follows:

  Unit 1   **Unit 2**   **Unit 3**
  MacAndrew   Elizabeth   D.
  MacDonald   Joseph
  MacHenry   Sharon   L.

- *Titles and seniority indicators either preceding or following a name should be disregarded. These are noted on the record only so that you can address the person properly. Thus Dr. Mary A. Smith and Henry R. Adams, Jr. are indexed as:*

Unit 1	Unit 2	Unit 3
Smith	*Mary*	*A. (Dr.)*
Adams	*Henry*	*R. (Jr.)*

- *Married women who have adopted their husband's surname are indexed using the woman's given name. For example, put the file under Mrs. Helen J. Smith, not Mrs. John C. Smith (Helen J.)*

- *Government offices are indexed by level of government. This is first stated by nationality, followed by department, bureau, and division, requiring additional units. This knowledge is used more often in locating information in a telephone directory. Thus the United States Justice Department, Bureau of Narcotics and Dangerous Drugs is indexed as:*

Unit 1	Unit 2	Unit 3	Unit 4
United	*States*	*Justice*	*Narcotics*

- *Banks are indexed by city, bank name, and state. Thus First Interstate of Tulsa is indexed as:*

Unit 1	Unit 2	Unit 3
Tulsa	*First Interstate*	*Oklahoma*

- *Person's surnames that can be mistaken for given names should be cross-indexed by placing an OUTguide or blank folder in the correct site. For example, John R. James should be properly indexed as follows:*

Unit 1	Unit 2	Unit 3
James	*John*	*R.*

  The mistaken site marker for this patient should read:

Unit 1	Unit 2	Unit 3	
John	*James*	*R.*	*SEE*
James	*John*	*R.*	

Record Safety

1. Do not leave files unattended on desks or counters.
2. Be sure that file drawers are closed when not in use.
3. When the office is closed, files should be locked to maintain confidentiality.
4. If your files are on computer, be sure that the computer is positioned so that only the operator may view the screen.
5. For security, use passwords to access individual files.

CHAPTER 11   Medical Office Management

Medical Office Management and Its Primary Purpose
The primary purpose of systems management is to achieve patient care and comfort by maintaining an efficient and effective medical practice. In the management of administrative systems, the Medical Administrative Assistant must be aware of the following principles:
- ✓ Each system is used in every medical practice or agency in varying degrees of complexity.
- ✓ The various systems are integrated and function simultaneously.
- ✓ The efficiency of each system depends on and affects all of the other systems.
- ✓ After each system has been planned, developed, and instituted, the medical administrative assistant observes, monitors, and evaluates the process for efficiency and effectiveness.

The Medical Administrative Assistant needs to develop an understanding of the elements of the following administrative systems: personnel management, communications (oral and written), appointment systems, records management, financial management, and facility and equipment management

Personnel Management
Solo Assistant Office.
1.   In a limited medical practice employing a single medical assistant, the physician/owner takes the role of manager and decision maker
2.   The medical administrative assistant is responsible for carrying out directives and maintaining all systems necessary for the efficient operation of the facility
3.   The assistant will be responsible for the duties of both front and back office.
Multiple-Employee Office.
- ✓ To allow the physician the freedom to concentrate on the primary goal of providing patient care, an office manager is hired.
- ✓ The office manager, in turn, coordinates the clinical and administrative staff duties necessary to promote total patient care.

Qualifications of an Office Manager
General qualities that are basic requirements for any manager include the following: objectivity, organizational skills, creativity, effective communication skills (written and oral), and diplomacy.

Communications Systems
An effective communication system is another vital component of medical office management. Communication systems include both oral and written communication. These systems should be thought of as key link between the physician and the patients. The impression made through communication reflects on all personnel and on the medical practice in general.

Scheduling Systems

An effective method of scheduling appointments is necessary for the efficient organization of the work involved in a health care facility. These appointment systems must be well developed since they affect all personnel and, most importantly, the patients who will be using the services provided by the health care facility.

Records Management

An efficient system of managing patient's medical records is essential for a well-run medical office. This includes structured systems for patient registration, preparing records, and handling and storing charts.

Financial Management

The management of financial systems in a facility involves the following three areas of responsibility:

- Billing systems
- Insurance
- Banking and Bookkeeping

Good financial management systems are essential to run a medical office. The income generated by billing and insurance provides the funds with which the practice or agency conducts business. One employee may be responsible for all financial records management, or the responsibility may be distributed among various staff members with specific skills who specialize in one or more aspects of the responsibility.

Facilities and Equipment Management

Facilities must be organized and maintained for maximum efficiency, and the equipment required to fulfill the various assisting responsibilities must be acquired and monitored. As a system for managing the facilities and equipment is developed, four basic factors must be considered: *patient comfort, accessibility of equipment and supplies, safety, and security.*

Office Security

Some areas of the office are considered high security; these are areas where narcotics, medications, and syringes are stored. Another high-risk area is where the staff members place their personal belongings. It is important that all areas have secure locks. You may consider consulting with a professional security service. It is important to have the areas around the building illuminated with sensor lights that have unbreakable shields. Alarms are helpful for security.

Before leaving the office each evening, all windows and doors should be double-checked. The physician who maintains controlled substances (narcotics) on the premises must keep these drugs in a locked cabinet or safe. Any loss of controlled substances by theft must be reported to the regional office of the Drug Enforcement Agency at the time the theft is discovered.

OSHA Requirements

The Occupational Safety and Health Administration (OSHA) issued safety standards in 1984 to handle gas sterilization in the medical office. Private physicians must provide nurses and other health care workers with protective clothing, vaccinations, and protection against–Bloodborne diseases such as AIDS and hepatitis B. Protective clothing or equipment includes gowns, latex gloves, mouth guards, and other protective gear.

Needlestick Safety and Prevention Act.

- Employers are required to involve employees in the selection of needle safety devices.
- The facility must be able to prove that consideration was given to various types of devices that promote needle safety, what led to the decision to choose the device currently in use, and which employees were involved in these decisions.
- A list should be kept of which employees contributed to the selection decisions.
- Minutes from meetings, copies of employee response forms, and the forms used to solicit are good methods of proving that employees were involved in the selection process
- A needlestick and sharps injury log must be kept in the medical facility.

CHAPTER 12   The Health and Accident Insurance

History of Insurance

1. Mid-1800s, insurance was first used for accidents to cover income loss rather than to cover expenses.
2. 1930s, medical insurance was generally used for hospital expenses and surgical/obstetrical procedures performed by physicians in hospitals.
3. 1929, Blue Cross was established in Texas when a group of schoolteachers made arrangements for prepaid hospital insurance with Baylor Hospital.
4. 1956, the government started CHAMPUS and Medicaid.
5. 1966, Medicare was established by the federal government to cover persons aged 65 and over, people with disabilities, and dependent widows.
6. 1980s, most people had indemnity plans that paid some or all of the expenses for covered services for illnesses or accidents for the policyholder and covered dependents. Benefits were decided on a fee-for-service basis, which means that they were based on what the physician charged for the services.
7. 1980s, more employers offered group insurance, which people began to use more frequently, causing health care costs to rise dramatically.

Insurance Basics

- Insurance is protection against financial loss caused by possible but unplanned events that can affect an individual or business.
- It can be acquired from:
  2. Private companies – e.g., Aetna and Travelers
  3. Government agencies – e.g. TRICARE (formerly CHAMPUS), CHAMPVA, Medicare, Medicaid, and Worker's Compensation.

Types of Insurance Plans

4. Private Plans

1. *Blue Cross/Blue Shield.*
   - Oldest indemnity plans.
   - They are non-profit community service organizations, although some have converted to for-profit status.
   - They assist federal and state governments in the administration of Medicare and Medicaid.
2. *Commercial carriers.*
   - These are private companies that enroll patients for premiums.
3. *HMOs.*
   - These are prepaid medical services and are either a closed panel HMO, which has its own facilities complete with physicians and services, or an open HMO, which contracts with physicians on a fixed-fee basis.

- Government Plans.
  - *TRICARE (formerly CHAMPUS).*
    - This program covers expenses for dependents of active-duty members of the uniformed services and for retired military personnel.
    - It also covers dependents of military personnel who were killed while on active duty.
      - *CHAMPVA.*
    - The Civilian Health and Medical Program of the Veterans Administration is for veterans with permanent service-related disabilities and their dependents.
    - It also covers surviving spouses and dependent children of veterans who died from service related disabilities.
      - *Medicare.*
    - Is a federal health plan that covers persons aged 65 and over, people with disabilities, and dependent widows.
      - *Medicaid.*
    - Covers low-income people who cannot afford medical care, which is cosponsored by federal and state governments.
    - Qualifications and benefits vary by state.
      - *Worker's Compensation.*
    - Covers people with job-related illnesses or injuries while benefits vary according to state law.
      - Premiums are the fees paid to a carrier to be protected by an insurance policy.
        1. Factors in determining premiums:
          - ✓ Likelihood that the insured will need financial reimbursement.
          - ✓ Likelihood that an event will occur.
          - ✓ Company's past experience with claims.
    - ✓ The policy is evaluated at the end of the period to determine if the premium should be adjusted.
    - ✓ Excessive claims against an insurance policy may result in an increase in an individual premium.
    - ✓ If the insured is part of the group, the cost of protection can be shared.

Insurance Benefits

- ✓ Helps patients to defray or reduce the amount of personal money that an individual must pay for health care services.
- ✓ Patient Responsibility.
  - ✓ Read their insurance plan literature and understand which services are covered by the insurance company.
3. Insurance Information Cards contains the following:
   - The carrier's name
   - The patient's name
   - The patient's group number and personal subscriber identification number
   - Where to submit claims
   - A brief description of covered services
   - Telephone number for prior authorization
- CMAA Responsibility.
  - Request to see the identification card of all insured patients at the time of the first visit and make a photocopy of the card, the front and back, for your record.
  - Verify periodically to recheck the patient's address, telephone number, and employment information.

Types and Components of Health and Accident Insurance

- Access to Health Insurance.
  - ✓ As individual, anyone with money who can pay the insurance premium can contract with a carrier for any insurance plan available.
  - ✓ As part of the Group, formed by people who work together or belong to the same labor union.
- Components of Health Insurance.
  - *Basic Benefits.*
    - ✓ Non-surgical services.
    - ✓ Laboratory and radiological diagnostic studies.
    - ✓ Does not cover routine physical examinations, eye examinations, family planning services, or medically necessary equipment such as artificial limbs.
    - ✓ Maximum annual benefit allowed.
  - ➢ *Major Medical Benefits.*
    1. Coverage begins where the basic plan leaves off such as hospitalization, surgery, radiation, or oncology treatment.
       - ✓ *Catastrophic Benefits.*
    - To cover long-term illnesses such as long-term recovery from a transplant or a long-term ailment where transplant may not be viable.
    - Coverage takes over when the major medical plan is maximized to its dollar limit, usually $1 million.
    - Assists in meeting expenses for inpatient services in an acute-care facility.
1. Supplemental Plans
   - Designed to pick up the payment of the 20% not paid by conventional insurance plans available to the patient or subscriber as a supplement to Medicare.

5. Special Automobile Insurance.
   - Covers injuries incurred as a result of vehicular accident.
- Insurance for the Medical Office.
   - Basic reason is to protect against financial loss
   - CMAA responsibilities are as follows:
   - Storing and retrieving policies.
   - Reminding the physician when the premium is due.
   - Establish a means to ensure that payment dates are not missed.
      - Classification of Insurance Policies.
   1. Property
   2. Criminal loss
   3. Disability
   4. Liability
   5. Life
   6. Overhead
   7. Bonding

Claim Insurance Process
1. File the insurance claim form, which identifies the policyholder or dependents and tells the insurance carrier which medical services were performed and why.
2. Certified Billing and Coding Specialist (CBCS) are responsible for processing insurance claim forms.
3. Five steps in the payment process of a patient's insurance claim form:
   - **Step 1** The patient completes (or updates) the patient information form.
   - **Step 2** The physician diagnoses and treats the patient and completes the encounter form.
   - **Step 3** The CBCS ensures that all codes are current then completes the claim form and submits it to the insurance carrier.
   - **Step 4** The insurance carrier processes the claim, makes appropriate payment, and provides an explanation of benefits.
   - **Step 5** The CBCS records payment and reviews the explanation of benefits for accuracy.

CHAPTER 13   Credit, Collections and Appeals

Importance of Accounts Receivable and the Responsibilities to the Billing System
8. Credit and Collection.
   a. Medical Administrative Assistants are responsible for maintaining accurate billing procedures and fee structures and collecting outstanding accounts receivable.
   b. Medical Administrative Assistants also are responsible for educating patients about specific charges on their statements and about the office policy on fee establishment, account collection, and credit.
9. Administrative Medical Assistant's Responsibilities.

a. *Responsibilities To Office in relation to the billing system are*: maintain accurate billing procedures and fee structures collect outstanding accounts receivable, and monitor constantly for potential breaks.

1. *Responsibilities To Patients:* educate the patient, which involves explaining specific items noted on individual statements, and should begin before medical services are provided, at which time the Administrative Medical Assistant can explain to each new patient the office policy on fee establishment, account collection, and credit.

i. Setting Fees - It requires understanding of the Resource-Based Relative Value Study (RBRVS) in addition to knowledge of "limiting charges" by the Health Care Financing Agency (HCFA) now known as CMS for Medicare reimbursement by geographical location. The RBRVS and the Federal Register provide the procedural code, a brief description, unit value, and days of follow-up if a CPT code is a surgical procedure.

- Physician Fee Profile.
  - A profile is a numerical image of a physician's patterns for charging for various services as monitored by insurance companies that are billed for reimbursement.
  - The individual profiles physicians refer to represent usual fees.
  - Comparative profiles are developed from all fees submitted by any physician in the geographical area for each service code.
  - These profiles set the standards for usual, customary, and reasonable (UCR) fees and determine the maximum charges an insurance carrier will allow.
- Usual Fees
  - Usual fees for each physician are calculated by computer and represent the fees routinely charged by a physician for each service.
  - To determine a physician's usual fee, select a specific time period (at least 1 year), and check the fees for a specific procedure at the various times throughout the year.
  - The fee that occurs most often is the usual fee.
  - For example, if your survey reveals charges for a specific procedure to include $10, $12, $12, $14, and $16, the usual fee would be $12.
- Customary Fees
  - ✓ Fees are considered customary if they fall within the upper and lower profile limits for physicians of the same specialty or practice type who practice within a geographical area determined by the insurance company.
  - ✓ If the upper limit profile is $18 for a specific service code and the lower limit is $14, the physician who submits a bill for $16 will have the fee recognized as customary.
- Reasonable Fees
  - Fees commonly are declared reasonable if they meet the criteria for usual and customary fees.

How to discuss fees with patients

- The assistant must listen to the patient's medical problem but should be prepared to discuss the expense, if the patient requests information about the fee.
- After the patient explains the medical problem, the assistant should tactfully inquire as to whether the patient has health insurance coverage.
- A patient should never be judged by his or her outward appearance.

- The rule is that the medical assistant must never assume anything about the patient's financial status.
- Fees for medical service should be stated clearly and a matter of fact.
- If a patient has a financial problem, the office manager in a separate room to avoid the embarrassment of discussing the issue in front of other people should interview the patient.
- The CMAA must be alert to certain signs that indicate that the patient may not choose to pay for services or treatment which include the following: no employment record, no home or work telephone number, a motel address, no referral, and no insurance.

4. It is best to ask the patient who cannot supply the above information to pay at time of service.

Credit and Collection Policies and Procedures
- Reasons For A Policy
    - ✓ Establishes guidelines for informing the patient of payment procedures.
    - ✓ Standardizes the information given by all employees to all patients.
    - ✓ Reduces the overall costs to all patients by avoiding the expense of repeated billing and possibly collection agency fees.

Aging of Accounts Receivable
Aging is a term applied to the technique of classifying each account with a balance due by the length of time the amount has been owed to the office. Aging segments are stated in terms of 30, 60, 90 and over 90 days, averaging all months out to 30 days each.

Computer Systems - It will produce an aging report for you on demand or request. In addition it can be sorted by insurance or patient so that there are no accounts left unpaid.

Account Age and Collectibility.

1. The longer an account exists without any payment being made on it, the less likely it is that the account will ever be collected.
2. Everyone is aware that each day a dollar is worth less than it was the day before.
3. Therefore each day that elapses until a bill is paid mean that, in the end less than the amount charged will actually be collected.
4. Accounts should be considered for beginning collection attention at approximately 45 days of aging, before the third statement.

Appeals Process

1. If a claim is denied and can be appealed; locate the appeals address on the back of the Explanation of Benefits.
2. Create an appeals letter using block letter format, including the following information: date inside address, recipient name, date of birth, insurance identification number, total charge, balance due and reason(s) that you do not agree with the decicion of the insurance company.
3. Send this letter immediately because the deadline for submitting an appeal will vary form payer to payer. Usually the timeframe is anywhere from (30-45 days).

CHAPTER 14 Computer Use In The Medical Practice

Basic Computer use in the Medical Practice

Just a few of the reasons for electing to computerize the office include the following:
- ✓ Office efficiency is increased.
- ✓ Overall cost is lower than with manual processing of information.
- ✓ Better management control and more current information will be available.
- ✓ The physician may expand the practice more conveniently.
- ✓ Collections may be improved.
- ✓ Records are more secure.

Types of Computers

1. Mainframe Computer - It is the largest of all computers. They are normally used in large facilities such as hospitals, centralized clinics operating with several outlying clinics, research institutes, and universities.
2. Laptop, Notebook, and Palmtop Computers - The smallest computers. They serve as portable personal computers meant for traveling either long distances or to local meetings or seminars.
3. Microcomputers - This is a desktop computer which has widely expanded uses and user-friendly applications for a multitude of business applications including the medical office
4. Minicomputers - These computers are frequently found in health care facilities since they normally have larger storage capacities.

Basic Components of the Computer

- • System Unit
- ✓ *Central Processing Unit (CPU)* - The brain of a computer; controls and coordinates the functions of all other components and processes information.
- • *Random Access Memory (RAM)* - Device that information temporarily for the applications being run; the individual applications are located into the RAM from the long-term storage device.
- • *Hard Drive* - The hard disk drive or hard drive is a feature that holds the computer's internal memory and can store a vast amount of information within the computer on a permanent basis, including both application and data storage.
- • *Removable Media Disk Drive* - A device that enables large amounts of information to be moved to and from the computer's hard drive from floppy (removable) disk or tape.
- • *CD-Rom Drive (Optional)* - A component that enables the computer to gain access to and use information available on a compact disk.
- • *Keyboard* - Letter and number pad similar to that of a typewriter and calculator combined that enables the user to input data and interact with the computer by typing in information or hitting special function keys.
- • *Mouse* - Device used to enter information into a computer by clicking on information or commands displayed on the monitor screen as well as selecting and moving data on screen; usually used in conjunction with the keyboard.
1. *Monitor* - Component similar to a television screen that allows the user to see what is occurring within the system at any given time.
2. *Printer* - It is an output device that prints the documents appearing on the monitor called printouts or hard copy.

3. *Removable Storage Devices* - It holds information just like a hard drive, but can easily be physically removed and taken to another location or computer.
4. *System Software* - Information used by the CPU to control the basic functions of the computer.
1. *Scanner-* Automated machine the reads and enters information from a document into the computer to prevent the need for typing large amounts of data; also can be used to copy images into the computer.
2. *Modem* - Device that converts data for transmission to the data processing equipment, usually from a telephone; the term comes by merging the terms modulator and demodulator.
1. *Computer Networks* - Often two or more computers may be connected to form a network. These computers may be in close proximity to each other and connected with special wiring, or they may be physically distant and connected over telephone lines. Being part of a network allows two or more computers to share the same information, resources, and printers, and increase productivity.
2. *Computer Service Systems* - An in-house or office computer system is made up of equipment – hardware, software, documentation, and data – that together perform an important task.

Application Software

- Word Processing.
  - Software program that allows the user to type and format documents.
- Spreadsheets.
  - Financial software program
1. Database Programs
     - Software designed to store and categorizes large amounts of similar information.
1. Billing Systems
     a. It is computerized billing software.

Security for data

1. The first step in records security is to verify the authenticity of all confidential medical and personal information as it is entered in to the database.
2. The second step is to implement security levels or passwords that permit only authorized individuals into the system.
3. Each specific security level permits access only to areas appropriate to that user's needs.
4. Procedures for adding or changing information on the database should indicate individuals authorized to make specific changes and time periods in which these changes will take place.
5. Passwords should be changed regularly, and the passwords for all terminated or former employees should be eliminated from the system.
6. If a practice uses a service bureau, all source documents, reports, and data should be returned to the practice when their contractual agreement is terminated.

CHAPTER 15   Banking

Basic Functions of Banking and the Medical Administrative Assistant's Responsibility for Interaction with the Bank

    A. The basic banking functions the Medical Administrative Assistant will encounter involve the following activities: *depositing funds, withdrawing funds, reconciling statements, and using auxiliary services.*

    B. Statements of the checking account are sent from the bank every month and must be reconciled immediately to verify the funds available to the practice.

    C. Checking - A check is a written order for the transfer of money.

    D. Reasons for writing checks.

    E. Checks are a safe method of paying out money.

    F. You can maintain a good record of the money.

    G. You will have good tax records.

    H. Money is protected while in the bank.

    I. You receive monthly summaries of your account.

    J. A "stop payment" option is available if you need the service.

    K. Checking Account Types.

    L. *Bank Checks, Cashier's Checks, Certified Checks, Limited Checks, and Voucher Checks.*

    A. Accepting Checks For Accounts Receivable

        A. Avoid accepting checks where the payer if unknown to you which are known as third-party checks, because the payee is the third person in the process.

        B. Because you do not have contact or experience with the payer, you increase the risk that the funds are not available to pay the face value of the check.

        C. Finally, checks with the notation "in full" or "paid in full" written on the face indicate that the patient understands that their account will have a zero balance once the check is recorded. You will need to be certain that this is correct before depositing the check.

    M. Endorsement of Checks A check must be endorsed to transfer the funds from one person to another which is accomplished by signing or rubber-stamping the back of the check in ink, at the left end, and perpendicular to the bottom of the check.

    N. The Uniform Negotiable Instrument Act regulates endorsements in all states.

    B. Problem Checks.

1. When a check is returned, a returned item notice will accompany it.

2. Before submitting a check to the bank, you should examine all entries on the face for completeness and accuracy.

3. Common errors include the following: date missing, payee's name missing, signature missing, and discrepancy between amount in numerals and amount written out.

   ° If the date or payee's name is missing, you may fill them in; if the signature is missing or the amounts do not match, the check must be returned to the payer.

   ° The bank also will reject a check that is not endorsed. Double-check the back of each to check to be certain that the item has been stamped or signed before you deposit it.

   ° The final reason the bank may return a check is difficulty with the payer which is something you cannot predict or prevent.

   ° Returned checks in this group will be stamped with an explanation, usually one of the following: *Refer to maker*- indicates that you should contact the payer for an explanation.

Non-sufficient funds (NSF)- indicates that the payer's account does not contain sufficient funds to pay the amount stated on the check *Others* – indicates that there may be problems such eligibility or a signature that does not match the one on file with the bank

1. Checks that are incomplete or include errors can be handled in several ways. You can return the check to the payer with an explanation and request a new check, advise the payer that you will hold the incorrect check until a replacement arrives, or advise the payer to bring a correct check on the next visit if it is within the next few days.

2. When a check is returned with a "Refer to Maker" or "NSF" notation, telephone the payer immediately. The payer may explain that an error was made and request that the check be resubmitted for payment. To accomplish this, cross out the notification stamp, write the word "resubmit" on the face and back of the check, and prepare a new deposit slip.

3. If you have any doubts about the credibility of the check or if the patient is relatively new to the practice and you do not have credit history, you may wish to pursue more aggressive collection measures. You may also check the office policy or practice for guidance.

General Policies about Deposits

When working with incoming funds, you should do the following:

A. Keep daily receipts in single, safe location.
B. Prepare and make deposits daily.
C. Compare the deposit slip total with the day sheet.
D. Keep duplicates of deposit slips in the office.
E. Keep bank receipts of deposits.
F. Record the deposit total in the checkbook or master calendar.

Check Writing Techniques

Method of Completing Checks.

1. Checks must be written with materials that cannot be altered.
2. They should be handwritten in ink or typewritten.
3. Another option is to write out all information except the net amount of the check, which may be imprinted by a machine that perforates the paper.
4. Complete the date, payee's name, check amount in numerals and handwriting, and memorandum portion with invoice numbers, if applicable.
5. Any supporting documents and the envelope in which the check will be mailed should be attached before presenting the check for signature.

Errors on Checks.

A. If a major error occurs when preparing a check such as writing the name of the payee on the line provided for the handwritten dollar amount, the check becomes invalid.
B. You will need to strike a line across the entire face of the check and, using ink, write the word "VOID" in large letters on it. The check is retained as proof of its invalid status.
C. If the error is minor, such as writing the number 74 when you intended to write 84, you may change the 7 to 8; the authorized signee must initial the change.

CHAPTER 16 Accounting and Bookkeeping

What is Accounting?

Accounting is an art of recording, classifying, and summarizing financial transactions.

Basic Bookkeeping Guidelines

A. Print letters and numbers correctly and legibly to decrease the possibility of errors.
B. Any entries in financial records must be made in ink, since they are permanent legal records.
C. When totaling columns, you may note the amounts in pencil until they are double-checked and you are certain that they balance.
D. Then you may super-impose the verified totals in ink.
E. If errors are noted after an entry has been made, they are corrected in the same manner as a medical record; you should strike through the error with a single line, without obliterating the entry, and insert the correct information.
F. Regardless of the type of bookkeeping system used, the following rules apply:
G. Fees and payments should be posted immediately.

H. Checks should be endorsed with a restrictive endorsement stamp as they are received.
I. Duplicate receipts should be prepared for all cash payments.
J. Deposits should be prepared daily.
K. All statements for accounts payable should be checked against invoices for accuracy and due date.
L. All financial transactions should be conducted by check.
M. A petty cash fund should be established, including the voucher system to account for expenditures

Types of Accounting Systems

A. *Single Entry* is a bookkeeping function in which each dollar amount charged for services, received as income, or paid out for services is recorded in only one place in the accounting records.

B. *Double* Entry - This bookkeeping system is more sophisticated because it is used by accountants to verify results and provide a built-in mechanism for the rapid identification of entry and computing errors. The fundamental principle of a double-entry system is that each entry to a debit account has a corresponding entry to a credit account and is based on the following equation:

$$Assets = Liabilities + Owners' Equity$$

A. *One-Write Pegboard Bookkeeping* also known as "write-it-once system" generates an entry on the day sheet at the same time that a check is written.

A. Computerized systems automatically post all of the journal entries for the accountant and provide a wide variety of reports such as profit and loss statements and balance sheets.

B. This system contains a payroll module, which is one of the most time saving portions of these programs.

C. Working inside the payables system, the payroll system calculates each employee's gross pay, plus all taxes and other deductions. It then writes the paycheck, records the transaction in the checking account, and keeps track of the tax liabilities. Do the calculations, the payroll system uses built-in tax tables, programmed by state.

Payroll

A. Payroll records are considered separately because of the legal directive involved in maintaining and reporting the information. When establishing a medical practice, each employer must apply for a federal and state employer's tax number that must be used on all forms and correspondence submitted to government agencies.

B. The first step in establishing a payroll record for each employee is the completion of a W4 form. The data submitted on the employee's W4 form are used to determine both federal and state withholding taxes.

C. Payroll accounting involves keeping a record of the gross salary, taxes withheld, and other deductions such as insurance or retirement contributions

Payroll Taxes

A. *Federal Income Tax*- Employers are required by law to withhold and process federal taxes for each employee.

B. *FICA Tax* - Several taxes commonly known as Social Security Tax are covered under the Federal Insurance Contribution Act (FICA). FICA is different from income tax in that every dollar contributed by an employee is matched by a dollar from the employer and the funds are used for individuals who are retired or unable to work.

C. *State Income Tax* - Some states have set up a mechanism similar to that of the federal government that allows employees to withhold a portion of each paycheck for deposit on estimated annual taxes due by employees.

D. *State Disability Insurance* - Some states have established funds to protect individuals temporarily unable to work because of illness or injury.

E. *Unemployment Insurance* - It is available in each state for individuals who have lost their jobs through unavoidable circumstances.

F. *Depositing Taxes Withheld* - Employers are required to deposit federal taxes they withheld to Federal Reserve Bank or authorized commercial bank on a monthly or quarterly basis.

G. Tax deposit forms are sent annually to each registered employer and must be submitted with each deposit.

H. The amount of the deposit equals the total accumulated federal income and FICA taxes withheld from employees and the matching FICA employer contribution.

I. Required Reports.

    J. For tax purposes the calendar year is divided into quarters, and the mandatory quarterly reports must be submitted on or before the last day of the month that follows the end of the quarter.

    K. Annual reports involve the preparation of the W-2 forms; these are six-part forms supplied by the federal government or purchased in most office supply stores.

    L. Because of their complexity, an accountant usually prepares employer's personal income taxes.

    M. Tax payments are made quarterly according to an estimate of the total amount due by the end of the year

    N. The final payment for the previous year must be submitted with the annual reports by April 15 of the present year and represent any amount due over the estimated payments already made.

BIBLIOGRAPHY

Eggers, De A., Conway, Anne M., *Mosby's Front Office Skills for the Medical Assistant*, St. Louis, Missouri: Mosby, Inc., 2000.

Young, Alexendra P., *KINN'S the Administrative Medical Assistant: an Applied Learning Approach*, Edition 5, St. Louis, Missouri.

Sample Test Questions 1

A. A medical administrative assistant's duties include all of the following, except:
1. Patient Reception
2. Money Management
3. Prepare the patient and equipment needed before the examination
4. Setting up appointments

B. The brain of the computer is the:
1. Hard disk
2. CPU
3. Memory
4. CRT

C. The least structured appointment system is:
1. Open Office Hours
2. Modified wave
3. Double booking
4. Time-specified

D. When patient failed to keep an appointment, the medical assistant should perform the following, except:
1. Record this information in the appointment book
2. Draw a line through the name of the patient and write the reason for the cancellation
3. Note n/s (for no-show) or f/s (failed to show) in the appointment book
4. Call and reprimand the patient

E. Registered mail provides the sender with:
1. Insurance protection
2. An inexpensive way to send valuables
3. Quick delivery
4. A receipt that must be retained until the item is received by the addressee

F. The amount owed by the Medical Office to individuals or other companies is called:
1. Assets
2. Liabilities
3. Accounts payable
4. Accounts receivable

G. The basic banking functions you will encounter as medical assistant involve the following, except:
1. Depositing funds
2. Withdrawing funds
3. Bank reconciliation
4. Making journal entries

H. The person making the check is the:
1. Payer
2. Payee
3. Endorser
4. Bank

I. All of the following are required in good communications with patients, except:
• Taking time to listen with patience and kindness
• Using positive nonverbal response such as warm smile
• Communicating clearly, without the use of a lot of "uhs" or "you know"
• Pretend to take notes of the details given by the patient

J. The system that controls breathing is the:
- Circulatory system
- Digestive system
- Respiratory system
- Nervous system

K. The directional term meaning "toward the back" is:
- Anterior
- Lateral
- Posterior
- Superior

L. A _____ is a physician who specializes in the study of the female reproductive system.
- Genealogist
- Gynecology
- Gynecologist
- Obstetrician

M. Which is not included in the right to Hospital Service under the Patient's Bill of Rights?
1. The patient has the right to expect that the hospital can provide needed services
2. After immediate needs are met, the patient may be transferred to another agency better equipped to handle the patient's problems and needs
3. The patient is informed of the reason for the transfer and of other alternatives
4. The patient is treated as a person and given kind and thoughtful care

N. The abbreviation for office visit is:
1. Of Vis
2. OVis
3. OTC
4. OV

O. Which is not included in the right to Refuse Treatment under the Patient's Bill of Rights?
1. The patient is informed of any rules and regulations applying to his or her conduct as a patient
2. The person can refuse treatment
3. The patient does not have to consent to each treatment or procedure recommended by the doctor.
4. The doctor must inform the patient of the risks to life and health involved in refusing the treatment

Sample Test Answers

1. C	6. C	11. C
2. B	7. D	12. C
3. A	8. A	13. D
4. D	9. D	14. D
5. D	10. C	15. A

Sample Test Questions 2

1. The payment method in which hospitals are paid based on the actual costs of treating each patient is _____.

   a. service reimbursement

   b. cost-based reimbursement

   c. per diem

   d. prospective payment system

2. The term used to describe the individual who is responsible to pay for medical services provided is _____.

   a. patient

   b. guarantor

   c. dependent

   d. None of the above.

3. Third party payers review a claim by putting the claim through a series of steps to decide whether it should be paid. This process is called _____.

   a. adjudication

   b. administration

   c. authorization

   d. validation

4. A report that can be printed with the patient accounting system to easily identify severely overdue accounts is called a(n) _____.

   a. aging report

   b. delinquency report

   c. hardship list

   d. old debt inventory

5. The payment method in which hospitals are paid a set rate per day is _____.

   a. cost-based reimbursement

   b. fee-for-service

   c. per diem

   d. prospective payment system

6. The most popular type of medical insurance plan is ____.

a. indemnity

b. managed care

c. high deductible

d. major medical

7. The next step after claims have been sent to payers is ____.

a. precertification

b. admission

c. appeal

d. follow-up

8. An office with more than how many employees should have one person designated as a supervisor or office manager?

a. One

b. Two

c. Three

d. Four

9. Which statement is *true* regarding how utilization review relates to medical necessity?

a. Utilization reviews are conducted to ensure services provided are medically necessary.

b. Utilization reviews are conducted to determine accurate payments.

c. Utilization reviews are conducted to identify activities involving fraud.

d. None of these is true.

10. Systems that capture and store each patient's clinical data electronically are called ____.

a. charge description masters

b. EOB systems

c. clean claim programs

d. electronic health records

Sample Test 2 Answers

1. B	5. C	9. A
2. B	6. B	10. D
3. A	7. D	
4. A	8. C	

PICA | | | | PICA

1. MEDICARE	MEDICAID	TRICARE CHAMPUS	CHAMPVA	GROUP HEALTH PLAN	FECA BLK LUNG	OTHER	1a. INSURED'S I.D. NUMBER (For Program in Item 1)
(Medicare #)	(Medicaid #)	(Sponsor's SSN)	(Member ID#)	(SSN or ID)	(SSN)	(ID)	

2. PATIENT'S NAME (Last Name, First Name, Middle Initial)

3. PATIENT'S BIRTH DATE MM DD YY — SEX M F

4. INSURED'S NAME (Last Name, First Name, Middle Initial)

5. PATIENT'S ADDRESS (No., Street)

6. PATIENT RELATIONSHIP TO INSURED — Self Spouse Child Other

7. INSURED'S ADDRESS (No., Street)

CITY — STATE

8. PATIENT STATUS — Single Married Other — Employed Full-Time Student Part-Time Student

CITY — STATE

ZIP CODE — TELEPHONE (Include Area Code) ( )

ZIP CODE — TELEPHONE (Include Area Code) ( )

9. OTHER INSURED'S NAME (Last Name, First Name, Middle Initial)

10. IS PATIENT'S CONDITION RELATED TO:

11. INSURED'S POLICY GROUP OR FECA NUMBER

a. OTHER INSURED'S POLICY OR GROUP NUMBER

a. EMPLOYMENT? (Current or Previous) YES NO

a. INSURED'S DATE OF BIRTH MM DD YY — SEX M F

b. OTHER INSURED'S DATE OF BIRTH MM DD YY — SEX M F

b. AUTO ACCIDENT? PLACE (State) YES NO

b. EMPLOYER'S NAME OR SCHOOL NAME

c. EMPLOYER'S NAME OR SCHOOL NAME

c. OTHER ACCIDENT? YES NO

c. INSURANCE PLAN NAME OR PROGRAM NAME

d. INSURANCE PLAN NAME OR PROGRAM NAME

10d. RESERVED FOR LOCAL USE

d. IS THERE ANOTHER HEALTH BENEFIT PLAN? YES NO If yes, return to and complete item 9 a-d.

READ BACK OF FORM BEFORE COMPLETING & SIGNING THIS FORM.
12. PATIENT'S OR AUTHORIZED PERSON'S SIGNATURE I authorize the release of any medical or other information necessary to process this claim. I also request payment of government benefits either to myself or to the party who accepts assignment below.

SIGNED _____ DATE _____

13. INSURED'S OR AUTHORIZED PERSON'S SIGNATURE I authorize payment of medical benefits to the undersigned physician or supplier for services described below.

SIGNED _____

14. DATE OF CURRENT: MM DD YY — ILLNESS (First symptom) OR INJURY (Accident) OR PREGNANCY(LMP)

15. IF PATIENT HAS HAD SAME OR SIMILAR ILLNESS. GIVE FIRST DATE MM DD YY

16. DATES PATIENT UNABLE TO WORK IN CURRENT OCCUPATION MM DD YY FROM TO MM DD YY

17. NAME OF REFERRING PROVIDER OR OTHER SOURCE

17a.
17b. NPI

18. HOSPITALIZATION DATES RELATED TO CURRENT SERVICES MM DD YY FROM TO MM DD YY

19. RESERVED FOR LOCAL USE

20. OUTSIDE LAB? YES NO — $ CHARGES

21. DIAGNOSIS OR NATURE OF ILLNESS OR INJURY (Relate Items 1, 2, 9 or 4 to Item 24E by Line)

1. ___.___
2. ___.___
3. ___.___
4. ___.___

22. MEDICAID RESUBMISSION CODE — ORIGINAL REF. NO.

23. PRIOR AUTHORIZATION NUMBER

24. A. DATE(S) OF SERVICE		B.	C.	D. PROCEDURES, SERVICES, OR SUPPLIES		E.	F.	G.	H.	I.	J.
From MM DD YY	To MM DD YY	PLACE OF SERVICE	EMG	(Explain Unusual Circumstances) CPT/HCPCS	MODIFIER	DIAGNOSIS POINTER	$ CHARGES	DAYS OR UNITS	EPSDT Family Plan	ID. QUAL.	RENDERING PROVIDER ID. #
1											NPI
2											NPI
3											NPI
4											NPI
5											NPI
6											NPI

25. FEDERAL TAX I.D. NUMBER — SSN EIN

26. PATIENT'S ACCOUNT NO.

27. ACCEPT ASSIGNMENT? (For govt. claims, see back) YES NO

28. TOTAL CHARGE $

29. AMOUNT PAID $

30. BALANCE DUE $

31. SIGNATURE OF PHYSICIAN OR SUPPLIER INCLUDING DEGREES OR CREDENTIALS (I certify that the statements on the reverse apply to this bill and are made a part thereof.)

SIGNED _____ DATE _____

32. SERVICE FACILITY LOCATION INFORMATION
a. b.

33. BILLING PROVIDER INFO & PH # ( )
a. b.

CARRIER

PATIENT AND INSURED INFORMATION

PHYSICIAN OR SUPPLIER INFORMATION

Promise

CMS-1500 Form Locator

Form Locator	Narrative Description/Explanation
1	**INSURANCE CARRIER SELECTION** – Enter **X** for Traditional Medicaid. **Required.**
1a	**INSURED'S I.D. NUMBER** (FOR PROGRAM IN ITEM 1) – Enter the member IHCP identification (RID) number. Must be 12 numeric digits. **Required.**
2	**PATIENT'S NAME** (Last Name, First Name, Middle Initial) – Provide the member's last name, first name, and middle initial obtained from the automated voice-response (AVR) system, electronic claim submission (ECS), Omni, or Web interChange verification. **Required.**
3	PATIENT'S BIRTH DATE – Enter the member's birth date in MMDDYY format. Optional. SEX – Enter an **X** in the appropriate box. Optional.
4	INSURED'S NAME (Last Name, First Name, Middle Initial) – Not applicable.
5	PATIENT'S ADDRESS (No., Street), CITY, STATE, ZIP CODE, TELEPHONE (include Area Code) – Enter the member's complete address information. Optional.
6	PATIENT RELATIONSHIP TO INSURED – Not applicable.
7	INSURED'S ADDRESS (No., Street), city, state, ZIP Code, telephone (include area code)– Not applicable.
8	PATIENT STATUS – Enter **X** the appropriate box. Optional.
9	**OTHER INSURED'S NAME** (Last Name, First Name, Middle Initial) – If other insurance is available, and the policyholder is other than the member shown in fields 1a and 2, enter the policyholder's name. **Required, if applicable.**
9a	**OTHER INSURED'S POLICY OR GROUP NUMBER** – If other insurance is available, and the policyholder is other than the member noted in fields 1a and 2, enter the policyholder's policy and group number. **Required, if applicable.**
9b	OTHER INSURED'S DATE OF BIRTH – If other insurance is available, and the policyholder is other than the member shown in field 1a and 2, enter the requested policyholder birth date in MMDDYY format. Optional. SEX – Enter **X** in the appropriate box. Optional.
9c	**EMPLOYER'S NAME OR SCHOOL NAME** – If other insurance is available, and the policyholder is other than the member shown in field 1a and 2, enter the requested policyholder information. **Required, if applicable.**

Form Locator	Narrative Description/Explanation
9d	**INSURANCE PLAN NAME OR PROGRAM NAME** – If other insurance is available, and the policyholder is other than the member shown in field 1a and 2, enter the policyholder's insurance plan name or program name information. **Required, if applicable.**
10	**IS PATIENT'S CONDITION RELATED TO** – Enter **X** in the appropriate box in each of the three categories. This information is needed for follow-up third party recovery actions. **Required, if applicable.**
10a	**EMPLOYMENT? (CURRENT OR PREVIOUS)** – Enter **X** in the appropriate box. **Required, if applicable.**
10b	**AUTO ACCIDENT?** – Enter **X** in the appropriate box. **Required, if applicable.** **PLACE (State)** – Enter the two-character state code. **Required, if applicable.**
10c	**OTHER ACCIDENT?** – Enter **X** in the appropriate box. **Required, if applicable.**
10d	RESERVED FOR LOCAL USE – Not applicable.
	Fields 11 and 11a through 11d are used to enter member insurance information.
11	**INSURED'S POLICY GROUP OR FECA NUMBER** – Enter the member's policy and group number of the other insurance. **Required, if applicable.**
11a	**INSURED'S DATE OF BIRTH** – Enter the member's birth date in MMDDYY format. **Required, if applicable.** **SEX** – Enter an **X** in the appropriate sex box. **Required, if applicable.**
11c	**INSURANCE PLAN NAME OR PROGRAM NAME** – Enter the member's insurance plan name or program name. **Required, if applicable.**
11b	**EMPLOYER'S NAME OR SCHOOL NAME** – Enter the re quested member information. **Required, if applicable.**
11d	**IS THERE ANOTHER HEALTH BENEFIT PLAN?** Enter **X** in the appropriate box. If the response is *Yes*, complete Fields 9a–9d. **Required, if applicable.**
12	PATIENT'S OR AUTHORIZED PERSON'S SIGNATURE – Not applicable.
13	INSURED'S OR AUTHORIZED PERSON'S SIGNATURE – Not applicable.
14	**DATE OF CURRENT ILLNESS** (First symptom date) **OR INJURY** (Accident date) **OR PREGNANCY (LMP date)** – Enter the date of the last menstrual period (LMP) for pregnancy-related services in MMDDYY format. **Required for payment for pregnancy-related services.**
15	IF PATIENT HAS HAD SAME OR SIMILAR ILLNESS, GIVE FIRST DATE – Enter date in MMDDYY format. Optional.
16	**DATES PATIENT UNABLE TO WORK IN CURRENT OCCUPATION** – If Field 10a is *Yes*, enter the applicable FROM and TO dates in a MMDDYY format. **Required, if applicable.**
17	**NAME OF REFERRING PROVIDER OR OTHER SOURCE** – Enter the name of the referring physician. **Required, if applicable.** For waiver related services, enter the provider name of the case manager. **Required for Medicaid *Select* PMP.** *The term* referring provider *includes those physicians primarily responsible for the authorization of treatment for lock-in or restricted card members.*

Form Locator	Narrative Description/Explanation
17a*	**ID NUMBER OF REFERRING PROVIDER, ORDERING PROVIDER OR OTHER SOURCE** The qualifier indicating what the number represents is reported in the first box of 17a. The ID number (IHCP provider number or taxonomy) is reported following the qualifier in the second box of 17a. **Required for Medicaid Select PMP.** **Qualifiers/ID Number to report to IHCP:** **1D** is the qualifier that applies to the IHCP provider number also called the LPI. The LPI includes nine numeric characters and one alpha character for the service location. Atypical providers are not required to report the NPI and will report their LPI. For example, certain transportation and waiver service providers. **ZZ** is the qualifier that applies to the provider taxonomy code. The taxonomy code includes 10 alpha-numeric characters. The taxonomy code is required when reporting an NPI.
17b*	**NPI** – Enter the 10-digit numeric NPI of the referring provider, ordering provider, or other source. **Required for all healthcare providers, except atypical providers as of May 23, 2007.**
18	**HOSPITALIZATION DATES RELATED TO CURRENT SERVICES** – Enter the requested FROM and TO dates in MMDDYY format. **Required, if applicable.**
19	**RESERVED FOR LOCAL USE** – Enter the *Medicaid Select* primary medical provider (PMP) two-digit alphanumeric certification code. **Required for *Medicaid Select* members when the physician rendering care is not the PMP or a physician in the PMP's group or a clinic.** *the PMP qualifier and ID number in 17a.*
20*	OUTSIDE LAB? – Not applicable. CHARGES – Not applicable.
21.1 to 21.4.	**DIAGNOSIS OR NATURE OF ILLNESS OR INJURY** – Complete Fields 21.1., 21.2., 21.3., and/or 21.4 to field 24E by detail line. Enter the ICD-9-CM diagnosis codes in priority order. A total of four codes can be entered. At least one diagnosis code is required for all claims except those for waiver, transportation, and medical equipment and supply services. **Required.**
22	MEDICAID RESUBMISSION CODE, ORIGINAL REF. NO. – Applicable for Medicare Part B crossover claims only. For crossover claims the combined total of the Medicare coinsurance, deductible, and psych reduction must be reported on the left side of field 22 under the heading *Code*. The Medicare paid amount (actual dollars received from Medicare) must be submitted in field 22 on the right side under the heading *Original Ref No*. **Required, if applicable.**
23	PRIOR AUTHORIZATION NUMBER – The prior authorization (PA) number is not required, but entry is recommended to assist in tracking services that require PA. Optional.

Date of service is the date the specific services were actually supplied, dispensed, or rendered to the patient.

For services requiring authorization, the FROM date of service cannot be prior to the date the service was authorized. The TO date of service cannot exceed the date the specific service was terminated.

Form Locator	Narrative Description/Explanation
24A to 24I* Top Half – Shaded Area	**NATIONAL DRUG CODE INFORMATION** – The shaded portion of fields 24A to 24I will be used to report NDC information. **Required as of July 1, 2007.** To report this information, begin at field 24A as follows: 1. Enter the NDC qualifier of N4 2. Enter the NDC 11-digit numeric code 3. Enter the drug description 4. Enter the NDC Unit qualifier • F2 – International Unit • GR – Gram • ML – Milliliter • UN – Unit 5. Enter the NDC Administered Amount in the format 9999.99
24A Bottom Half	**DATE OF SERVICE** – Provide the FROM and TO dates in MMDDYY format. Up to six FROM and TO dates are allowed per form. **Required.**
24B	**PLACE OF SERVICE** – Use the POS code for the facility where services were rendered. **Required.** For a complete listing of POS codes, go to http://cms.hhs.gov/MedHCPCSGenInfo/Downloads/ Place_of_Serice.pdf.
24C*	**EMG** – Emergency indicator. This field indicates services were for emergency care for service lines with a CPT® or HCPCS code in field 24D. Enter **Y** or **N**. **Required, if applicable.**
24D	**PROCEDURES, SERVICES, OR SUPPLIES** **CPT/HCPCS** – Use the appropriate procedure code for the service rendered. Only one procedure code is provided on each claim form service line. **Required.** **MODIFIER** – Use the appropriate modifier, if applicable. Up to four modifiers are allowed for each procedure code. **Required, if applicable.**
24E	**DIAGNOSIS CODE** – Enter number 1–4 corresponding to the applicable diagnosis codes in field 21. A minimum of one and a maximum of four diagnosis code references can be entered on each line. **Required.**
24F	**$ CHARGES** – Enter the total amount charged for the procedure performed, based on the number of units indicated in field 24G. The charged amount is the sum of the total units multiplied by the single unit charge. Each line is computed independently of other lines. This is a ten digit numeric field. **Required.**
24G	**DAYS OR UNITS** – Provide the number of units being claimed for the procedure code. Six digits are allowed, and 9999.99 units is the maximum that can be submitted. The procedure code may be submitted in partial units, if applicable. **Required.**
24H	**EPSDT Family Plan** – If the patient is pregnant, indicate with a **P** in this field on each applicable line. **Required, if applicable.**

Form Locator	Narrative Description/Explanation
24I* Top Half - Shaded Area	**RENDERING ID QUALIFIER** – Enter the *Qualifier* indicating what the number reported in the shaded area of 24J represents. Either 1D for IHCP rendering provider number or ZZ for rendering provider taxonomy code **Required.** **Qualifiers or ID number to report to IHCP:** **1D** is the qualifier that applies to the IHCP provider number (LPI). The LPI includes nine numeric characters and one alpha character for the service location. Atypical providers are not required to report the NPI and will report their LPI. For example, certain transportation and waiver service providers. **ZZ** is the qualifier that applies to the provider taxonomy code. The taxonomy code includes 10 alpha-numeric characters. The taxonomy code is required when reporting an NPI.
24J* Top Half – Shaded Area	**RENDERING PROVIDER ID** – Enter either the LPI if entering the 1D qualifier in 24I or the taxonomy if entering the ZZ qualifier in 24I for the Rendering Provider ID. **Required, if applicable.** **LPI** – The entire nine-digit LPI must be used. If billing for case management, the case manager's number must be entered here. If billing for mid-level practitioners, the supervising physician's rendering provider number must be entered here. **Taxonomy** – Enter the taxonomy code of the rendering provider if you are entering the NPI in the bottom half of 24J.
24 J* Bottom Half	**RENDERING PROVIDER NPI** – Enter the NPI of the rendering provider. **Required if applicable.**
25	FEDERAL TAX I.D. NUMBER – Not applicable.
26	PATIENT'S ACCOUNT NO. – Enter the internal patient tracking number. Optional.
27	ACCEPT ASSIGNMENT? – The *IHCP Provider Agreement* includes details about accepting payment for services. Optional.
28	**TOTAL CHARGE** – Enter the total of all service line charges in column 24F. This is a 10-digit field, such as 99999999.99. **Required.**
29	**AMOUNT PAID** – Enter the payment received from any other source, excluding the 8A deductible and the Medicare paid amount. All applicable items are combined and the total entered in this field. This is a 10-digit field. **Required, if applicable.** Other insurance – Enter the amount paid by the other insurer. If the other insurer was billed but paid zero, enter **0** in this field. Attach denials to the claim form when submitting the claim for adjudication.
30	**BALANCE DUE** – TOTAL CHARGE (Field 28) – AMOUNT PAID (Field 29) = BALANCE DUE (Field 30). This is a 10-digit field, such as 99999999.99. **Required.**
31	**SIGNATURE OF PHYSICIAN OR SUPPLIER INCLUDING DEGREES OR CREDENTIALS** – An authorized person, someone designated by the agency or organization, must sign and date the claim. A signature stamp is acceptable; however, a typed name is not. Providers who have signed the *Signature on File* certification form will have their claims processed when a signature is omitted from this field. The form is available on the IHCP Web site, *Provider Services* page at http://www.indianamedicaid.com/ihcp/ProviderServices/provider_enroll.asp. **Required if applicable.** **DATE** – Enter the date the claim was filed. **Required.**
32*	SERVICE FACILITY LOCATION INFORMATION – Enter the provider's name and address where the services were rendered, if other than home or office. This field is optional, but it helps EDS contact the provider, if necessary. Optional.
32a*	SERVICE FACILITY LOCATION NPI – Not applicable.

Form Locator	Narrative Description/Explanation
32b*	SERVICE FACILITY LOCATION QUALIFIER AND ID NUMBER – Not applicable.
33*	BILLING PROVIDER INFO & PH # – Enter the billing provider service location name, address, and the expanded ZIP Code + 4 format. Required. Note: If the U.S. Postal Service provides an expanded ZIP Code for a geographic area, this expanded ZIP Code must be entered on the claim form.
33a*	BILLING PROVIDER NPI – Enter the billing provider NPI. Required, if applicable.
33b*	BILLING PROVIDER QUALIFIER AND ID NUMBER – Enter a billing provider qualifier of ZZ and taxonomy code for a NPI. If the billing provider is an atypical provider, enter the qualifier 1D and the LPI. Required. During the transition period, billing provider may report the qualifier 1D and the LPI. Note: Qualifiers are ZZ = Taxonomy and 1D = IHCP provider number (LPI)

Note: These instructions apply to the IHCP guidelines only and are not intended to replace instructions issued by the NUCC. The NUCC instruction manual can be found at http://www.nucc.org.

An example of the claim form is included.

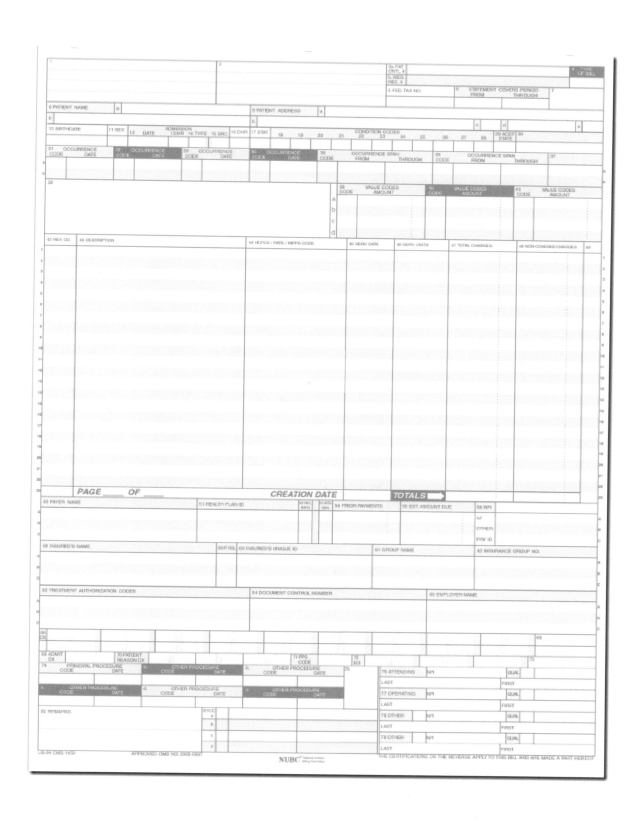

UB-04 data field requirements

1 Provider Name and Address Required Required	2 Pay-To Name and Address Situational Situational
3a Patient Control Number Required Required	3b Medical Record Number Situational Situational
4 Type of Bill Required Required	5 Federal Tax Number Required Required
6 Statement Covers Period Required Required	7 Future Use N/A N/A
8a Patient ID Situational Situational	8b Patient Name Required Required
9 Patient Address Required Required	10 Patient Birthdate Required Required
11 Patient Sex Required Required	12 Admission Date Required Required, if applicable
13 Admission Hour Required Required, if applicable	14 Type of Admission/Visit Required Required
15 Source of Admission Required Required	16 Discharge Hour Required N/A
17 Patient Discharge Status Required Required	18-28 Condition Codes Required, if applicable Required, if applicable
29 Accident State Situational Situational	30 Future Use N/A N/A
31-34 Occurrence Codes and Dates Required, if applicable Required, if applicable	35-36 Occurrence Span Codes and Dates Required, if applicable Required, if applicable
37 Future Use N/A N/A	38 Responsible Party Name and Address Required, if applicable Required, if applicable
39-41 Value Codes and Amounts Required, if applicable Required, if applicable	42 Revenue Code Required Required
43 Revenue Code Description Required Required NDC Code Required, if applicable Required, if applicable 29 Accident State Situational Situational	30 Future Use N/A N/A
31-34 Occurrence Codes and Dates Required, if applicable Required, if applicable	35-36 Occurrence Span Codes and Dates Required, if applicable Required, if applicable
37 Future Use N/A N/A	38 Responsible Party Name and Address Required, if applicable Required, if applicable
39-41 Value Codes and Amounts Required, if applicable Required, if applicable	42 Revenue Code Required Required
43 Revenue Code Description Required Required	NDC Code Required, if applicable Required, if applicable 35-36 Occurrence Span Codes and Dates Required, if applicable Required, if applicable
37 Future Use N/A N/A	38 Responsible Party Name and Address Required, if applicable Required, if applicable
39-41 Value Codes and Amounts Required, if applicable Required, if applicable	42 Revenue Code Required Required
43 Revenue Code Description Required Required	NDC Code Required, if applicable Required, if applicable
44 HCPCS/Rates Required, if applicable Required, if applicable	45 Service Date N/A Required
46 Units of Service Required Required	47 Total Charges (By Rev. Code) Required Required
48 Non-Covered Charges Required, if applicable Required, if applicable	49 Future Use N/A N/A
50 Payer Identification (Name) Required Required	51 Health Plan Identification Number Situational Situational
52 Release of Info Certification Required Required	53 Assignment of Benefit Certification Required Required
54 Prior Payments Required, if applicable Required, if applicable	55 Estimated Amount Due Required Required

56 NPI Required Required	57 Other Provider IDs Optional Optional
58 Insured's Name Required Required	59 Patient's Relation to the Insured Required Required
60 Insured's Unique ID Required Required	61 Insured Group Name Situational Situational
62 Insured Group Number Situational Situational	63 Treatment Authorization Codes Required, if applicable Required, if applicable
64 Document Control Number Situational Situational	65 Employer Name Situational Situational
66 Diagnosis/Procedure Code Qualifier Required, if applicable Required, if applicable	67Principal Diagnosis Code/Other Diagnosis
Codes	Required Required
68 Future Use N/A N/A	69 Admitting Diagnosis Code Required Required, if applicable
70 Patient's Reason for Visit Code Situational Situational	71 PPS Code Situational Situational
72 External Cause of Injury Code Situational Situational	73 Future Use N/A N/A
74 Principal Procedure Code/Date Required, if applicable Required, if applicable	75 Future Use N/A N/A
76 Attending Name/ID-Qualifier 1G Required Required	77 Operating ID Situational Situational
78-79 Other ID Situational Situational	80 Remarks Situational Situational
81 Code-Code Field/Qualifiers	*0-A0 N/A N/A
*A1-A4 Situational Situational	*A5-AB N/A N/A
AC - Attachment Control number Situational Situational	AD-B0 N/A N/A
*B1-B2 Situational Situational	*B3 Required Required

An example of the claim form is included.

Blue Cross UB04 Form Locator

UB-04 Claim Form Instructions
FORM LOCATOR NAME INSTRUCTIONS

1. Billing Provider Name &
Address
Enter the name and address of the hospital/facility
submitting the claim.

2. Pay to Address Pay to address if different than field 1.

3a. Patient Control Number Enter your facility's unique account number
assigned to the patient, up to 20 alpha/numeric
characters. This number will be printed on the RA
and will help you identify the patient.

3b. Medical Record Number Number assigned to patient's medical record by provider. Up to 30 alpha/numeric characters.

4. Type of Bill Enter the four digit code that identifies the specific type of bill and frequency of submission. The first digit is a leading zero.

2nd Digit - Submitting Facility

1 = Hospital
2 = Skilled Nursing
3 = Home Health
4 = Christian Science (Hospital)
5 = Christian Science (Extended Care)
6 = Intermediate Care
7 = Clinic (Use "2nd Digit - Clinics Only" below)
8 = Special Facility (Use "2nd Digit - Special Facilities Only" below)

2nd Digit - Bill Classification (*Except Clinics and Special Facilities*)

1 = Inpatient (Including Medicare Part A)
2 = Inpatient (Medicare Part B Only)
3 = Outpatient
4 = Other
5 = Intermediate Care - Level I
6 = Intermediate Care - Level II
7 = Intermediate Care - Level III
8 = Swing Beds

2nd Digit - Clinics Only

1 = Rural Health
2 = Hospital Based or Independent Renal Dialysis Center
3 = Free Standing
4 = Outpatient Rehabilitation Facility (ORF)
5 = Comprehensive Outpatient Rehabilitation Facility (CORF)
9 = Other

2nd Digit - Special Facilities Only

1 = Hospice (Non-Hospital Based)
2 = Hospice (Hospital Based)
3 = Ambulatory Surgery Center
4 = Free Standing Birthing Center
9 = Other

3rd Digit - Frequency

0 = Non-Payment/Zero Claim
1 = Admit Through Discharge Date (one claim covers entire stay)
2 = First Interim Claim
3 = Continuing Interim Claim

4 = Last Interim Claim

5 = Late Charge(s) Only Claim

6 =

7 = Replacement of Prior Claim

8 = Void/Cancel of Prior Claim

5. Federal Tax Number Enter the facility's tax identification number.

6. Statement Covers Period Enter the beginning and ending service dates of
for the period covered on the claim in MMDDYY
format.

7. Administrative Necessary Days Enter the number of Administratively Necessary
Days (AND).

8. Patient Name Enter the recipient's name exactly as it is spelled
on the Medical Assistance ID card.

9. Patient Address Enter the recipient's mailing address including
street address, city, state and zip code.

10. Birth Date Enter the recipient's date of birth in MMDDCCYY
format.

11. Sex Enter "M" for Male, "F" for Female or "U" for
unknown.

12. Admission Date Enter the start date of this episode of care. Use the
MMDDCCYY format.

13. Admission Hour Enter the hour (using a two-digit code below) that
the patient entered the facility.
1:00 a.m. - 01 2:00 a.m. - 02
3:00 a.m. - 03 4:00 a.m. - 04
5:00 a.m. - 05 6:00 a.m. - 06
7:00 a.m. - 07 8:00 a.m. - 08
9:00 a.m. - 09 10:00 a.m. - 10
11:00 a.m. - 11 12:00 noon - 12
1:00 p.m. - 13 2:00 p.m. - 14
3:00 p.m. - 15 4:00 p.m. - 16
5:00 p.m. - 17 6:00 p.m. - 18
7:00 p.m. - 19 8:00 p.m. - 20
9:00 p.m. - 21 10:00 p.m. - 22
11:00 p.m. - 23 12:00 a.m. - 24/00

14. Admit Type Enter one of the following primary reason for
admission codes:
1 = Emergency
2 = Urgent
3 = Elective
4 = Newborn
5 = Trauma
9 = Information Not Available

15. Source of Admission Enter one of the following source of admission
codes:
1 = Physician Referral
2 = Clinic Referral
3 = HMO Referral
4 = Transfer from Hospital
5 = Transfer from SNF
6 = Transfer From Another Health Care Facility
7 = Emergency Room
8 = Court/Law Enforcement
9 = Information Not Available
In the Case of Newborn
1 = Normal Delivery
2 = Premature Delivery
3 = Sick Baby
4 = Extramural Birth

16. Discharge Hour Enter the hour (using a two-digit code below) that
the patient entered the facility.
1:00 a.m. - 01 2:00 a.m. - 02
3:00 a.m. - 03 4:00 a.m. - 04
5:00 a.m. - 05 6:00 a.m. - 06
7:00 a.m. - 07 8:00 a.m. - 08
9:00 a.m. - 09 10:00 a.m. - 10
11:00 a.m. - 11 12:00 noon - 12
1:00 p.m. - 13 2:00 p.m. - 14
3:00 p.m. - 15 4:00 p.m. - 16
5:00 p.m. - 17 6:00 p.m. - 18
7:00 p.m. - 19 8:00 p.m. - 20
9:00 p.m. - 21 10:00 p.m. - 22
11:00 p.m. - 23 12:00 a.m. - 24/00

17. Patient Discharge Status Enter one of the following two-digit codes for the patient's status (as of the "through" date):

01 = Discharged to home or self care (routine discharge)

02 = Discharged/transferred to another short-term general hospital

03 = Discharged/transferred to skilled nursing facility (SNF)

04 = Discharged/transferred to an intermediate care facility (ICF)

05 = Discharged/transferred to another type of institution

06 = Discharged/transferred to home under care of organized home health service organization

07 = Left against medical advice

08 = Reserved

09 = Admitted as an inpatient to this hospital (Medicare Outpatient Only)

20 = Expired (or did not recover - Christian Science patient)

21 – 29 Reserved

30 = Still a patient

40 = Expired at home

41 = Expired in a medical facility; e.g., hospital, SNF, ICF, or free-standing hospice (Medicare Hospice Care Only)

42 = Expired - place unknown (Medicare Hospice Care Only)

43 = Discharged to Federal Health Care Facility

50 = Hospice- Home

51 = Hospice – Medical Facility

52- 60 Reserved

61 = Discharge to Hospital Based Swing Bed

62 = Discharged to Inpatient Rehab

63 = Discharged to Long Term Care Hospital

64 = Discharged to Nursing Facility

65 = Discharged to Psychiatric Hospital

66 = Discharged to Critical Access Hospital

18-28. Condition Codes Enter two digit alpha numeric codes up to eleven occurrences to identify conditions that may affect processing of this claim. See National Uniform Billing Committee for guidelines.

29. Accident State Enter two-digit state abbreviation.

30. Accident Date Date accident occurred.

31-34. Occurrence Codes and
Dates
Enter up to four code(s) and associated date(s) for
any significant event(s) that may affect processing
of this claim.
01 = Auto Accident
02 = Auto Accident - No Fault Insurance
03 = Accident - Tort Liability
04 = Accident - Employment Related
05 = Other Accident
06 = Crime Victim
09 = Start of Infertility Treatment
11 = Illness - Onset of Symptoms
12 = Date of Onset For Chronically Dependant
16 = Date of Last Therapy
17 = Date Outpatient Occupational Therapy
18 = Date of Retirement
20 = Date Guarantee of Payment Began
21 = Date UR Notice Received
22 = Date Active Care Ended
24 = Date Insurance Denied
25 = Date Benefits Terminated By Primary Payer
26 = Date Skilled SNF Became Available
27 = Date Hospice Certification
28 = Date Comprehensive Outpatient Rehab
29 = Date Outpatient Physical Therapy
30 = Date Outpatient Speech Pathology
31 = Date Beneficiary Notified of Intent to Bill
(procedures)
32 = Date Beneficiary Notified of Intent to Bill
33 = First Day of COB for ESRD
34 = Date of Election of Extended Care
35 = Date Treatment for Physical Therapy
36 = Date of Inpatient Discharge for Covered
Transplant
37 = Date of Inpatient for Non-Covered
Transplant
38 = Date Treatment for Home IV
39 = Date Discharged on Continuous IV
40 = Scheduled Date of Admission
41 = Date of First Test Pre-Admit
42 = Date of Discharge
43 = Cancelled Surgery
44 = Inpatient Admit Changed to Outpatient

44 = Date Treatment Started Occupational
45 = Date Treatment Started Speech
46 = Date Treatment Started Cardiac Rehab
47 = Date Cost Outlier Begins
A1= Birth Date- Insured A
A2 = Effective Date – Insured A Policy
A3 = Benefits Exhausted
A4 = Split Bill Date
B1= Birth Date-Insured B
B2 = Effective Date Policy B
B3 = Benefits Exhausted – Payer B
C1 = Birth Date – Insured C
C2 = Effective Date – Insured C
C3 = Benefits Exhausted -Payer C

35-36. Occurrence Span Enter the span of occurrence dates as indicated in 31 - 35.

38. Responsible Party Name and
Address
Enter the responsible party name and address.

39. - 41. Value Code and Amount Enter up to three value codes to identify special circumstances that may affect processing of this
claim. See NUBC manual for specific codes.
In the Amount box, enter the number, amount, or
UCR value associated with that code.

42. Revenue Code Enter a four digit Revenue Code beside each
service described in column 43.
(See Section 800, "Revenue Codes.")
After the last Revenue Code, enter "0001"
corresponding with the Total Charges amount in
column 47. (PAPER CLAIMS ONLY)

43. Description Enter a brief description that corresponds to the
Revenue Code in column 42. List applicable
NDC if location 44 is a J code.
Report the N4 qualifier in the first two (2)
positions, left justified, followed immediately by
the 11 character NDC number. Immediately
following the last character of the NDC (no space)
the Unit of Measurement Qualifier immediately

followed by the quantity with a floating decimal
with a limit of 3 characters to the right of the
decimal point.
Unit of Measurement:
F2 - International Unit
GR - Gram
ML - Milliliter
UN - Unit
To report more than one NDC per HCPC use the
NDC attachment form.
Enter "Total Charges" after the last description in
this column to correspond with the total of all
charges amount in column 47.

44. HCPC Utilized for outpatient bills. If billing for an
injectable code must display an NDC in location
43.

45. Service Date Enter the date this service was provided
(MMDDCCYY format).

46. Service Units Enter the number of hospital accommodation days
or units of service (such as pints of blood) which
were rendered. AND days must correspond to the
number of days in form locator 7.

47. Total Charges Enter the total amount charged for each line of
service. Also, enter the total of all charges after
the last amount in this column.

48. Non-Covered Charges Enter the amount, if any that is not covered by the
primary payer for this service.

50. Payer Enter the name and three-digit carrier code of the
primary payer on line A and other payers on lines
B and C. (Medical Assistance is always the payer
of last resort.)
**If the patient has Medical Assistance only,
enter "RI Medicaid" on line A.**
If Medicare is the primary payer, indicate Part A
or Part B coverage.

51. Health Plan ID The number used by the health plan to identify
itself.

52. Release of Information Enter "Y" for yes or "N" for no.

53. Assignment of Benefits Enter "Y" for yes.

54. Prior Payments Enter the amounts paid by the other insurance
payers listed in form locator 50. If payment is
made by other insurance, proof of payment (e.g.,
EOB) must be attached to the claim form.

55. Estimated Amount Due The amount estimated to be due.

56. National Provider Identifier
Billing Provider (NPI)
Unique identifier assigned to the provider. Seven
digit RI Medical Assistance Provider ID if not
submitting NPI.

57. Other Provider Identifier **Taxonomy must be entered if NPI is entered in
location 56**. This id **must** be entered in line A,B,C
that corresponds to the line in which the "RI
Medicaid" payer information is entered in locator
50.

58. Insured's Name If other health insurance is involved, enter the
insured's name.

59. Patient's Relation to Insured Enter the code for the patient's relationship to the
insured.
01 = Spouse
18 = Self
19= Child
20 = Employee
21 = Unknown
39 = Organ Donor
40 = Cadaver Donor
53 = Life Partner
G8 = Other Relationship

60. Insured's Unique Identifier Enter recipient's nine-digit Medical Assistance ID.
This id **must** be entered in line A,B,C that
corresponds to the line in which the RI Medicaid
payer information is entered in locator 50.

61. Group Name Enter the name of insured's other group health
coverage, if applicable.

62. Insurance Group Number Enter insured's group number, if applicable.

63. Treatment Authorization
Number
Number that designates that treatment has been
authorized.

64. Document Control Number Control number assigned to the original bill.

65. Employer Name Name of employer providing health coverage.

66. Diagnosis and Procedure Code
Qualifier
Enter 9 for ICD 9 coding.

67. Principal Diagnosis Code on
Admission
Enter the ICD-9-CM diagnosis code that describes
the nature of the illness or injury.

67A - Q Other Diagnosis Codes Enter up to 16 ICD-9-CM codes for other
diagnoses.

68. Admitting Diagnosis Code Enter the ICD-9-CM diagnosis code that describes
the patient's condition at the time of admission.

70. Patient's Reason for Visit Enter the ICD-9-CM diagnosis code that describes
the patient's reason for visit..

71. PPS Code The PPS code assigned to the claim.

72. External Cause of Injury Code Enter the ICD-9-CM diagnosis code pertaining to
external cause of injuries.

74. Principal Procedure Code and
Date
Enter the ICD code that identifies the principal
procedure performed. Enter the date of that
procedure.

74A-E. Other Procedure Codes Enter other ICD codes identifying all significant
procedures performed. Enter the date of those
procedures.

76. Attending Provider Name and
Identifiers

Enter NPI of individual in charge of patient care.
If UPIN number is entered, qualifier must be 1G.
Enter the last and first name below.

77. Operating Physician Name and
Identifiers
Required when surgical procedure is performed.
Enter the NPI. If UPIN number is entered,
qualifier must be 1G. Enter the last and first
name.

78. - 79. Other Provider Name and
Identifiers
Enter the NPI. If UPIN number is entered,
qualifier must be 1G. Enter the last and first
name.

80. Remarks Field/**Signature Enter provider signature or authorized agent.**
81cc. Code-Code Field Enter B3 in the qualifier if locations 76-79 contain
an NPI. **Enter the corresponding provider
taxonomy of provider NPI's entered in
locations**
76a – 81CCa
77b – 81CCb
78c – 81CCc
79d – 81CCd

Exam 1

True/False
Indicate whether the statement is true or false.

_____ 1. Job responsibilities of the medical assistant include executing banking responsibilities.

_____ 2. The medical assistant is not responsible for following directions if an emergency arises.

_____ 3. Assertiveness involves being pushy and overbearing.

_____ 4. Physical demands of the administrative medical assistant may include performing library research and typing manuscripts.

_____ 5. Kübler-Ross's stages of dying consistently occur in the order described in this chapter.

_____ 6. A hospice program offers medical care and support to patients and family members dealing with a terminal illness and loss of a loved one.

_____ 7. A career in health care is very desirable because there is a very low level of stress.

_____ 8. Certification for any health care professional is controlled by the government.

_____ 9. Family practices offer comprehensive medical care for individuals of all ages.

_____ 10. It is important for an administrative medical assistant in the field of pediatrics to like elderly people and have a background in aging.

_____ 11. It is important for an administrative medical assistant in the field of psychiatry to know the skeletal and muscular anatomy and disease and terminology.

_____ 12. An administrative medical assistant in the field of plastic surgery should be skilled in obtaining accurate, detailed case histories.

_____ 13. Radiology involves treatment, diagnosis, and prevention of diseases by x-rays and radium.

_____ 14. Managed care organizations operate under the concept of prepaid group health care.

_____ 15. The specialized approach to health care evolved from the philosophy that the physical, mental, and social well-being of the "whole" person is as important as the treatment of a separate medical problem.

_____ 16. The Oath of Medicine of today is based on the Oath of Caduceus.

_____ 17. Ethical principles should be reflected in administrative procedures.

_____ 18. The principles adopted by the AMA are laws.

_____ 19. The medical professional has long subscribed to a body of ethical statements developed primarily for the benefit of the physician.

_____ 20. It is appropriate for a medical assistant to make critical statements about the treatment given a patient by another physician.

_____ 21. Once a physician is licensed in one state, she may practice medicine in all states.

_____ 22. A medical assistant cannot be sued.

_____ 23. Litigation is trial by jury following a plaintiff's filing of a complaint or petition.

_____ 24. Protected health information (PHI) is any information about the patient's health condition that contains personal identifying data.

_____ 25. HIPAA only deals with rules that guarantee confidentiality and privacy.

_____ 26. Communication is the transfer of information from one party to another.

_____ 27. Negative communication could affect diagnosis and treatment.

_____ 28. Good communicators focus only on themselves.

_____ 29. Basic, or physiologic needs, such as food, water, air, and sleep, must be met before moving on to other types of needs.

_____ 30. Always use very technical language when speaking to the patient.

_____ 31. Nonverbal communication is conscious and intentional.

_____ 32. The body language of a patient usually depicts their true feelings and emotional state.

_____ 33. Change the subject if you become uncomfortable with a patient who is conveying his feelings.

_____ 34. A child will often base his opinion on his past experiences and what he has been told by his parents.

_____ 35. The medical assistant should be aware of factors that vary from culture to culture when communicating with others.

_____ 36. Rudeness is acceptable if you are in a hurry.

_____ 37. In the medical office, it is important to address the physician with the title "doctor" unless told otherwise.

_____ 38. When asked to do something new, the medical assistant should respond "that is not in my job description."

_____ 39. Avoid gossip, arguments, and uncomplimentary statements about coworkers.

_____ 40. When listening to a speech-impaired patient, it is okay to pretend to understand.

Multiple Choice
Identify the choice that best completes the statement or answers the question.

_____ 41. A professional attitude involves
   a. confidence.
   b. responsibility.
   c. empathy.
   d. all of the above.

_____ 42. The heart of the health care professional involves
   a. stress and burnout.
   b. empathy and service.
   c. burnout and anxiety.
   d. skill and education.

_____ 43. In the next five to ten years, health care careers will
   a. grow by 10%.
   b. not grow.
   c. double.
   d. grow up to 60%.

_____ 44. Being able to put yourself in the patient's situation is an important skill called
   a. empathy.
   b. demeanor.
   c. sympathy.
   d. integrity.

_____ 45. What is the first stage of dying, which appears to be a defense mechanism and may recur at other times during the dying process?
   a. Anger
   b. Depression
   c. Denial
   d. Bargaining

_____ 46. During which stage of dying may the patient try to keep information private, so others may or may not be aware of any problem?
   a. Acceptance
   b. Depression
   c. Denial
   d. Bargaining

_____ 47. Credentialing that is sanctioned and required by a state's government is called
   a. certification.
   b. accreditation.
   c. registration.
   d. licensure.

_____ 48. What type of knowledge is vital in avoiding medical professional liability suits?
   a. Medicolegal
   b. Computer
   c. Technical
   d. Interpersonal

_____ 49. What are two good indicators of job satisfaction?
   a. Empathy and sympathy
   b. Initiative and motivation
   c. Pessimism and aggression
   d. Stress and burnout

_____ 50. To effectively counteract the effects of stress and burnout, the medical assistant should
   a. avoid interpersonal communication.
   b. treat patients as if they are interruptions.
   c. never vary office duties.
   d. exercise regularly.

_____ 51. What are two important tools in evaluating a patient's behavior?
   a. Sensitivity and commitment
   b. Listening and observing
   c. Assertion and concern
   d. Humor and consideration

_____ 52. Being friendly, sensitive, warm, genuine, courteous, and positive are signs of a medical assistant with good
   a. organizational skills.
   b. clinical skills.
   c. interpersonal skills.
   d. secretarial skills.

_____ 53. Who was the founder of the American Red Cross?
   a. Marie Curie
   b. Christiaan Barnard
   c. Clara Barton
   d. Louis Pasteur

_____ 54. Who is the founder of nursing?
   a. Clara Barton
   b. Florence Nightingale
   c. Marie Curie
   d. Jonas Salk

_____ 55. Who is the "father of medicine"?
   a. Hippocrates
   b. Aesculapius
   c. Imhotep
   d. Caduceus

_____ 56. In what type of practice do two or more practitioners share office expenses, employees, and the on-call schedule?
   a. Associate
   b. Group
   c. Solo physician
   d. Specialty

_____ 57. In what type of practice is the physician either on call 24 hours a day or shares calls with an independent practitioner?
   a. Group
   b. Professional corporation
   c. Solo
   d. Associate

_____ 58. What are most private, for-profit centers called that employ salaried physicians who compete directly with private physician practices?

    a. Urgent care centers   c. Hospitals

    b. Clinics   d. Laboratories

_____ 59. Which practice setting has several surgical suites and a delivery room in addition to an outpatient or same-day surgery unit?

    a. Urgent care center   c. Hospital

    b. Clinic   d. Group practice

_____ 60. In which practice setting can patients be admitted for special studies and treatment by a group of health care professionals practicing medicine together?

    a. Urgent care center   c. Hospital

    b. Laboratory   d. Clinic

_____ 61. What type of hospital treats the severely ill or injured patient?

    a. Acute care   c. Mental health

    b. Specialty   d. Convalescent

_____ 62. What type of hospital takes care of patients with psychiatric problems?

    a. Acute care   c. Mental health

    b. Specialty   d. Rehabilitation

_____ 63. What type of hospital provides 24-hour care for patients who have been declared medically stable, but who need acute and subacute rehabilitation?

    a. Convalescent   c. Rehabilitation

    b. Substance abuse   d. Specialty

_____ 64. What type of hospital are skilled nursing facilities an example of?

    a. Convalescent   c. Rehabilitation

    b. Substance abuse   d. Mental health

_____ 65. What specialty would best serve an elderly adult patient?

    a. Pediatrics   c. Gynecology

    b. Gerontology   d. Neurology

_____ 66. Intentional torts

    a. must be committed with force.

    b. are common in the medical field.

    c. are generally not covered by standard medical malpractice insurance policies.

    d. are caused by negligence.

_____ 67. Unintentional torts include

    a. assault and battery.

    b. breach of confidential communication.

    c. negligence.

    d. fraud.

_____ 68. What may be used in the physician's defense when the patient understood the risks of a particular operation or other medical procedure and signed a document giving informed consent?

    a. Assumption of risk   c. Statute of limitations

    b. Contributory negligence   d. None of the above

_____ 69. What mechanism is used when the patient and physician have agreed before treatment (preclaim agreement) that both will waive the right to a court trial in case of a dispute?

a. No-fault insurance
b. Arbitration
c. A screening panel
d. Litigation

70. When a direct verbal or written statement is used, what type of medical contract is it?
    a. Compliant
    b. Implied
    c. Terminated
    d. Expressed

71. Which of the following statements regarding minors is accurate?
    a. Each state has a different age of majority.
    b. Twenty-one is the majority age in all states.
    c. A parent must authorize any type of surgery or treatment in writing for a child in all the states.
    d. An 8-year-old child can authorize her own surgery or treatment.

72. When treating minors, it is advisable to
    a. discourage minors from involving their parents in medical decisions that are of a sensitive nature.
    b. seek parental approval in all cases.
    c. seek parental approval in cases that are not sensitive or confidential.
    d. not treat minors, it only brings trouble.

73. When a physician terminates supervision of a patient without notifying the patient in writing, it is known as
    a. informed consent.
    b. emergency care.
    c. abandonment.
    d. statute of limitations

74. What must be obtained and signed in order to disclose protected health information?
    a. Letter
    b. Fraud statement
    c. Power of attorney
    d. Authorization form

75. A document that allows an individual to delegate to another person the legal authority to act on her behalf is known as a/an
    a. expert testimony.
    b. deposition.
    c. durable power of attorney.
    d. living will.

76. What type of document allows patients to specify what they would and would not want done in four specific dire situations by checking forty-eight boxes?
    a. Medical directive
    b. Living will
    c. Durable power of attorney
    d. Consent form

77. Which of the following is considered an emancipated minor?
    a. A minor who is on active military duty.
    b. A minor who is married or divorced.
    c. A minor who becomes a parent.
    d. All of the above.

78. What act provides for the gifting of body parts to be used for transplant, research, or placement in a tissue bank after the death of an adult?
    a. Do Not Resuscitate Act
    b. Uniform Anatomical Give Act
    c. Advance Directive Act
    d. Medical Directive Act

79. The majority of human messages are communicated by
    a. body language.
    b. tonality.
    c. spoken word.
    d. feedback.

80. The value we place on ourselves and the need to be respected are
    a. safety needs.
    c. esteem needs.

b. self-actualization needs.   d. physiologic needs.

_____ 81. A patient who is visually impaired
     a. may need instructions written down.
     b. may need help filling out forms.
     c. should not be physically guided.
     d. will pay attention mainly to your body language.

_____ 82. Individuals who have an impaired level of understanding
     a. should be ignored.
     b. will require you to speak louder than you usually do.
     c. should be cared for with dignity.
     d. depend on lip-reading skills to understand.

_____ 83. When dealing with an anxious patient,
     a. acknowledge the patient's feelings of anxiety.
     b. belittle the patient's feelings of anxiety.
     c. ignore the patient's feelings of anxiety.
     d. none of the above.

_____ 84. Any patient with special needs should be treated with
     a. dignity.   c. caring.
     b. respect.   d. all of the above.

_____ 85. Leaning forward, making eye contact, and giving your full attention to the speaker is
     a. paraphrasing.   c. active listening.
     b. open ended.   d. defensive.

_____ 86. Communication can be affected by
     a. age.   c. economic status.
     b. gender.   d. all of the above.

_____ 87. When communicating with others, it is important to remember
     a. that body language is not important.
     b. not to interrupt others when they are speaking.
     c. everyone will react the same to what you say.
     d. to stand very close to the person when speaking.

_____ 88. Offering a toy or puppet may help in getting cooperation from
     a. adolescents.   c. children.
     b. older adults.   d. non-English speakers.

_____ 89. Which of the following is a soft response that may help calm a patient?
     a. I don't know!
     b. That's a difficult one. Let's see what we can do.
     c. We can't do that!
     d. Both a and c.

_____ 90. When dealing with an angry patient, the medical assistant should
     a. not take it personally.   c. maintain eye contact with the patient.
     b. remain calm.   d. all of the above.

Matching

Match each term with the correct statement below.

a. accreditation
b. administrative medical assistant
c. aggressive
d. assertive
e. burnout
f. certification
g. clinical medical assistant
h. continuing education units
i. empathy
j. flextime
k. hospice
l. interpersonal skills
m. stress
n. sympathy

_____ 91. a front-office medical assistant who performs secretarial duties
_____ 92. a system that allows employees to choose their own times for starting and finishing work within a broad range of available hours
_____ 93. forward, pushy, and overbearing behavior
_____ 94. putting yourself in the other person's situation
_____ 95. a back-office medical assistant who performs clinical and laboratory duties
_____ 96. liking people and getting along with others
_____ 97. a team that offers medical care and support for terminally ill patients and their family members
_____ 98. a way of tracking education that is pursued by a working professional and is intended to improve or maintain professional competence
_____ 99. a display of feelings that may actually inhibit your ability to help
_____ 100. the process of meeting a state standard or being evaluated and recognized by a national organization as meeting predetermined standards
_____ 101. a condition of physical, psychological, and emotional reactions to circumstances that causes strain, tension, and pressure
_____ 102. behavior that is confident, shows leadership, and resolves conflict peacefully
_____ 103. a condition that results from too much or too little stress

Match each term with the correct statement below.

a. clinic
b. group practice
c. hospital
d. laboratory
e. medical center
f. minute clinic
g. multispecialty practice
h. partnership
i. professional corporation
j. solo physician practice
k. specialized care center
l. urgent care center

_____ 104. facility offering medical services at sites other than a hospital setting
_____ 105. entity unto itself with a legal and business status that is independent of its shareholders
_____ 106. facility where a team of specialists treat patients who have similar medical conditions
_____ 107. facility where research, experimentation, and the physical and clinical analysis of specimens are performed
_____ 108. one physician working alone whose charges are based on a fee-for-service arrangement
_____ 109. group of physicians practicing at the same location, each specializing in a different field of medicine
_____ 110. facility that provides 24-hour care and treatment for the acutely sick and injured
_____ 111. two or more physicians practicing medicine under a legal partnership agreement that specifies the responsibilities, rights, and obligations of each entity
_____ 112. three or more physicians sharing office space, expenses, and so on

_____113. medical facility that may include several physicians of the same or different specialty where patients undergo examination and treatment

_____114. freestanding emergency centers, usually with extended evening and weekend hours

_____115. small clinic, usually found in small-scale chain store, offering limited services

Match each term with the correct statement below.

a. Dermatology	j. Orthopedics
b. Emergency Medicine	k. Otolaryngology
c. Gerontology	l. Pathology
d. Gynecology	m. Pediatrics
e. Internal Medicine	n. Physiatry
f. Neonatology	o. Podiatry
g. Neurology	p. Psychiatry
h. Obstetrics	q. Surgery
i. Ophthalmology	r. Urology

_____116. specialty dealing with treatment, diagnosis, and prevention of mental disorders

_____117. specialty providing consultations on and diagnosis of complex diseases

_____118. specialty dealing with disorders of the genitourinary tract

_____119. specialty dealing with disorders of the nervous system

_____120. specialty dealing with disorders of the skin

_____121. specialty dealing with treatment by operation

_____122. specialty dealing with treatment of trauma and sudden emergent conditions

_____123. specialty dealing with disorders of the eye and vision

_____124. specialty dealing with disorders of the ears and throat

_____125. specialty dealing with physical medicine and rehabilitation

_____126. specialty dealing with treatment of the musculoskeletal system

_____127. specialty dealing with the medical care of women during pregnancy and childbirth

Match each term with the correct statement below.

a. caduceus	g. independent practice association (IPA)
b. capitation	h. managed care organization (MCO)
c. continuing education unit	i. point of service (POS) plan
d. exclusive provider organization (EPO)	j. preferred provider organization (PPO)
e. fee-for-service (FFS)	k. primary care physician (PCP)
f. health maintenance organization (HMO)	l. utilization review

_____128. method of payment listing charges for services rendered

_____129. fixed fee paid monthly per enrolled patient, regardless of the amount of services actually used

_____130. managed care plan offering choice at the time services are needed of receiving services from an HMO, PPO, or fee-for-service plan

_____131. symbol of the medical profession (winged staff with two snakes)

_____132. process for monitoring and controlling medical testing and procedures, helping to curb health care costs

_____133. variation of the HMO where patients receive better benefits when going to participating physicians

_____134. measurement of time spent in professional development activity

_____135. exclusive large employers contract with limited physician network

_____136. group of individual providers who contract with an HMO or PPO but still see private patients

_____137. oldest form of prepaid health plan

_____138. health care delivery system that strives to manage cost, quality, and delivery of health care by emphasizing preventive medicine

_____139. physician with ongoing responsibility for overall treatment of a patient

Match each term with the correct statement below.

a. advance directive	h. defendant
b. authorization form	i. deposition
c. bioethics	j. emancipation
d. civil law	k. ethics
e. complaint	l. etiquette
f. compliance	m. expert testimony
g. consent form	

_____140. testimony of a witness under oath and written down before trial for possible use when the case comes to trial

_____141. branch of ethics dealing with issues arising in biomedical research

_____142. a statute that enforces private rights and liabilities

_____143. the first pleading of the plaintiff in a civil action

_____144. a person sued

_____145. a statement given concerning some scientific, technical, or professional matter by an expert

_____146. when signed by the patient, allows disclosure of health information

_____147. principles that are reflected in administrative procedures

_____148. the act of releasing or freeing

_____149. customary code of conduct, courtesy, and manners

_____150. patients can be denied treatment if they refuse to sign this form

_____151. form that details procedures to be performed or withheld when death is imminent

_____152. act of adhering to laws, rules, recommendations

Match each term with the correct statement below.

a. grievance committee
b. health care power of attorney
c. Health Insurance Portability and Accountability Act
d. implied consent
e. litigation
f. living will
g. plaintiff
h. privileged information
i. protected health information
j. respondeat superior
k. subpoena
l. subpoena duces tecum

m. tort

_____153. a confidential exchange between a professional and a client or patient, not to be disclosed without specific consent
_____154. one who institutes a lawsuit or action
_____155. "under penalty"
_____156. a private wrong or injury to a person that is grounds for legal action
_____157. any health information that contains personal identifying data
_____158. let the master answer
_____159. 1996 federal law dealing in part with confidentiality issues
_____160. not expressed by direct words but gathered by implication of the situation
_____161. legally binding document that allows an individual to detail precise wishes about treatment

Match each term with the correct statement below.

a. active listening	f. defensive
b. bias	g. demeanor
c. colloquialisms	h. discrimination
d. communicate	i. displaced anger
e. communication cycle	j. ethnic

_____162. transfer information from one party to another
_____163. exchange process involving sender, receiver, message, channel, and feedback
_____164. behavior that is unconscious and a response to protect oneself from a perceived threat
_____165. unfair treatment of an individual or group
_____166. being patient and giving the speaker your full attention
_____167. the person's appearance, expressions, and body language
_____168. one-sided opinion
_____169. slang or informal language
_____170. racial or cultural influences

Match each concept with the correct statement below.

a. enunciate	f. perceptions
b. feedback	g. prejudice
c. noncompliant	h. reflective listening
d. nonverbal communication	i. stereotyping
e. open-ended questions	j. verbal communication

_____171. judgment formed prior to gathering facts
_____172. sending a message without words
_____173. holding an attitude that all people from the same country are the same
_____174. pronounce clearly
_____175. awareness or assumptions that people make based on their point of view
_____176. the use of language or spoken words to transmit messages
_____177. providing feedback, which can be verbal or nonverbal, after listening
_____178. refusing to follow the doctor's instructions or plan
_____179. encourage patients to talk more

_____180. a verbal or nonverbal response

Completion
Complete each statement.

181. _____ is the process by which an agency or organization evaluates and recognizes a program of study or an institution as meeting certain predetermined standards.

182. Elisabeth Kübler-Ross explained five typical stages that a patient with a terminal illness may experience. They are _____, _____, _____, _____, and _____.

183. _____ was a term used in the Middle Ages to signify a place where weary pilgrims could stop and rest, but today it is a movement that helps terminally ill patients and their families.

184. Maintaining a/an _____ attitude will help the medical assistant avoid some of the negative consequences of stress.

185. A medical assistant will need to be competent in both _____ and _____ job skills in order to pass the American Association of Medical Assistants certification test.

186. _____ is an image you project by how you present yourself and how you conduct yourself as a health care worker.

187. Some of the resources available to a medical assistant to help adapt to change and keep up with current technology and practices are _____ _____, _____ _____, _____ _____, and _____ _____ _____.

188. As a certified or registered medical assistant, it will be necessary for you to obtain _____ on a regular basis.

189. "Think with _____, act through _____."

190. A vibrant medical practice is a/an _____-oriented practice, and this should be demonstrated by all who work there.

191. An understanding of medical _____ is an important skill for the medical assistant to communicate properly.

192. Being a medical assistant is more than a job–it is a/an _____.

193. To prevent misleading the patient unintentionally, good _____ _____ skills are necessary.

194. The _____ _____ _____ begins: "I believe in the principles and purposes of the profession of medical assisting."

195. "I will never learn how to do that" is an example of a/an _____ attitude.

196. Hospitals can be either _____ -owned or _____ -owned.

197. General and community hospitals are usually _____ and serve a specific geographical area and need in the community.

198. _____ hospitals, also called <u>private</u> or <u>investor-owned</u> hospitals, are controlled by the individual, partnership, or corporations that own them.

199. Hospital sizes are measured by the number of _____ provided with state licenses issued on that basis.

200. Physicians apply for _____ _____ at the hospitals of their choice.

201. A hospital's _____ department deals with insurance verification and precertification of insurance.

202. A hospital's _____ _____ department handles radioactive materials used in tests such as bone and liver scans.

203. Hospitals may be named for the type of _____ they serve.

204. When one is applying for a hospital position, it is wise to emphasize _____.

205. Today, ancillary or auxiliary services many hospitals offer are referred to as _____ services.

206. The name _____ _____ written after a hospital name usually denotes services provided at sites other than the hospital setting.

207. _____ can be independent, free-standing, or in a medical facility.

208. _____ _____ centers exist to serve the needs of a group of patients having similar medical conditions.

209. Physicians are very dependent on laboratory results to expedite the _____ and _____ of their patients.

210. Employment in a laboratory requires _____ and _____.

211. In a malpractice case, usually the physician is the _____.

212. The branch of study resulting from high technology and sophisticated biomedical research centering on moral issues, questions, and problems that arise in the practice of medicine is known as _____.

213. The Oath of Hippocrates set down the first standards of _____ _____ and _____.

214. Physicians graduating from medical school take the Oath of Hippocrates or the more modern oath called _____ _____ _____.

215. In 1980, the American Medical Association (AMA) adopted a modern code of ethics called the

_____ _____ _____ _____.

216. According to the AMA principles, a physician may ethically receive payments from patients for medical services but cannot accept a/an _____ of any kind from anyone.

217. Office _____ should be printed in a booklet or handout so that patients will be informed about charges for missed appointments, telephone calls, insurance form completion, and so forth.

218. Remember that everything seen, heard, or read about a patient is _____ and does not leave the office.

219. The customary code of conduct, courtesy, and manners in the medical profession is known as _____ _____.

220. Physical, verbal, or nonverbal sexual harassment in the workplace should be reported to a/an _____ or _____.

221. By the early 1900s, all the states had passed Medical Practice Acts because of the prevalence of _____.

222. The two types of medical professional liability insurance are _____ _____ insurance and _____ _____, or occurrence insurance.

223. _____ _____ is Latin for "Let the master answer."

224. An impartial panel established to listen to and investigate patients' complaints about medical care or excessive fees is known as a/an _____ _____.

225. _____ _____ _____ is a type of subpoena that requires a witness to appear in court with records, although sometimes the judge permits mailing of records, and the witness then need not appear.

226. Being patient while the message is spoken and giving the speaker your undivided attention involves _____ _____.

227. The most expressive part of the body is the _____.

228. _____ is a belligerent, combative attitude and is a type of defense mechanism.

229. Trying to maintain eye contact with someone who is uncomfortable may be perceived as aggression and create a communication _____.

230. The medical assistant should avoid _____ patients and should provide the same quality of service regardless of the patient's age, sex, race, and so forth.

231. A patient may become _____, refusing to follow the doctor's treatment plan.

232. Restating, or _____, tells the patient that you have listened and helps clarify what was said.

233. Asking _____ questions will help you bring forth information from patients.

234. Rather than agreeing or disagreeing with a patient's thoughts, ideas, or perceptions, it is better to remain _____ so the patient cannot conclude that you think they are right or wrong.

235. The _____ _____ includes the sender, message, channel, receiver, and feedback.

236. When communicating with a patient who is _____ impaired, it may be helpful to sit on their good side and use gestures.

237. A patient who is anxious about going to the doctor may have a reaction called

_____ _____.

238. Have a positive _____ in all your work assignments.

239. Maslow's _____ _____ _____ states that people are motivated by needs and that their basic needs must be met before they can progress to fulfill other needs.

240. Making up a reason to justify unacceptable actions, behaviors, or events is a defense mechanism called _____.

Short Answer

241. Instead of complaining about problems, how should the administrative medical assistant deal with problems?

242. Describe why an effective health care worker should be skilled at understanding human behavior.

243. What type of lifestyle is the patient encouraged to develop through the holistic approach to health care?

244. Is it necessary for the administrative medical assistant to be familiar with the abbreviations of medical positions? Why or why not?

245. Why was a Patient's Bill of Rights developed by the House of Delegates of the American Hospital Association?

246. List five instances when minors are considered emancipated.

247. List the five components of Maslow's hierarchy of needs in order of importance.

248. List five different types of defense mechanisms.

249. Briefly describe two differences between good communicators and poor communicators.

250. List three methods of providing feedback, either by oral or nonverbal response.

Exam 1
Answer Section

TRUE/FALSE

1.	ANS: T	PTS:	1
2.	ANS: F	PTS:	1
3.	ANS: F	PTS:	1
4.	ANS: T	PTS:	1
5.	ANS: F	PTS:	1
6.	ANS: T	PTS:	1
7.	ANS: F	PTS:	1
8.	ANS: F	PTS:	1
9.	ANS: T	PTS:	1
10.	ANS: F	PTS:	1
11.	ANS: T	PTS:	1
12.	ANS: T	PTS:	1
13.	ANS: F	PTS:	1
14.	ANS: T	PTS:	1
15.	ANS: F	PTS:	1
16.	ANS: F	PTS:	1
17.	ANS: T	PTS:	1
18.	ANS: F	PTS:	1
19.	ANS: F	PTS:	1
20.	ANS: F	PTS:	1
21.	ANS: F	PTS:	1
22.	ANS: F	PTS:	1
23.	ANS: T	PTS:	1
24.	ANS: T	PTS:	1
25.	ANS: F	PTS:	1
26.	ANS: T	PTS:	1
27.	ANS: T	PTS:	1
28.	ANS: F	PTS:	1
29.	ANS: T	PTS:	1
30.	ANS: F	PTS:	1
31.	ANS: F	PTS:	1
32.	ANS: T	PTS:	1
33.	ANS: F	PTS:	1
34.	ANS: T	PTS:	1
35.	ANS: T	PTS:	1
36.	ANS: F	PTS:	1
37.	ANS: T	PTS:	1

38.	ANS: F	PTS: 1
39.	ANS: T	PTS: 1
40.	ANS: F	PTS: 1

MULTIPLE CHOICE

41.	ANS: D	PTS: 1
42.	ANS: B	PTS: 1
43.	ANS: D	PTS: 1
44.	ANS: A	PTS: 1
45.	ANS: C	PTS: 1
46.	ANS: D	PTS: 1
47.	ANS: D	PTS: 1
48.	ANS: A	PTS: 1
49.	ANS: B	PTS: 1
50.	ANS: D	PTS: 1
51.	ANS: B	PTS: 1
52.	ANS: C	PTS: 1
53.	ANS: C	PTS: 1
54.	ANS: B	PTS: 1
55.	ANS: A	PTS: 1
56.	ANS: A	PTS: 1
57.	ANS: C	PTS: 1
58.	ANS: A	PTS: 1
59.	ANS: C	PTS: 1
60.	ANS: C	PTS: 1
61.	ANS: A	PTS: 1
62.	ANS: C	PTS: 1
63.	ANS: C	PTS: 1
64.	ANS: A	PTS: 1
65.	ANS: B	PTS: 1
66.	ANS: C	PTS: 1
67.	ANS: C	PTS: 1
68.	ANS: A	PTS: 1
69.	ANS: B	PTS: 1
70.	ANS: D	PTS: 1
71.	ANS: A	PTS: 1
72.	ANS: C	PTS: 1
73.	ANS: C	PTS: 1
74.	ANS: D	PTS: 1
75.	ANS: C	PTS: 1
76.	ANS: A	PTS: 1
77.	ANS: D	PTS: 1

78. ANS: B   PTS: 1
79. ANS: A   PTS: 1
80. ANS: C   PTS: 1
81. ANS: B   PTS: 1
82. ANS: C   PTS: 1
83. ANS: A   PTS: 1
84. ANS: D   PTS: 1
85. ANS: C   PTS: 1
86. ANS: D   PTS: 1
87. ANS: B   PTS: 1
88. ANS: C   PTS: 1
89. ANS: B   PTS: 1
90. ANS: D   PTS: 1

MATCHING

91. ANS: B   PTS: 1
92. ANS: J   PTS: 1
93. ANS: C   PTS: 1
94. ANS: I   PTS: 1
95. ANS: G   PTS: 1
96. ANS: L   PTS: 1
97. ANS: K   PTS: 1
98. ANS: H   PTS: 1
99. ANS: N   PTS: 1
100. ANS: A   PTS: 1
101. ANS: M   PTS: 1
102. ANS: D   PTS: 1
103. ANS: E   PTS: 1

104. ANS: E   PTS: 1
105. ANS: I   PTS: 1
106. ANS: K   PTS: 1
107. ANS: D   PTS: 1
108. ANS: J   PTS: 1
109. ANS: G   PTS: 1
110. ANS: C   PTS: 1
111. ANS: H   PTS: 1
112. ANS: B   PTS: 1
113. ANS: A   PTS: 1
114. ANS: L   PTS: 1
115. ANS: F   PTS: 1

116. ANS: P   PTS: 1
117. ANS: E   PTS: 1
118. ANS: R   PTS: 1
119. ANS: G   PTS: 1
120. ANS: A   PTS: 1
121. ANS: Q   PTS: 1
122. ANS: B   PTS: 1
123. ANS: I   PTS: 1
124. ANS: K   PTS: 1
125. ANS: N   PTS: 1
126. ANS: J   PTS: 1
127. ANS: H   PTS: 1

128. ANS: E   PTS: 1
129. ANS: B   PTS: 1
130. ANS: I   PTS: 1
131. ANS: A   PTS: 1
132. ANS: L   PTS: 1
133. ANS: J   PTS: 1
134. ANS: C   PTS: 1
135. ANS: D   PTS: 1
136. ANS: G   PTS: 1
137. ANS: F   PTS: 1
138. ANS: H   PTS: 1
139. ANS: K   PTS: 1

140. ANS: I   PTS: 1
141. ANS: C   PTS: 1
142. ANS: D   PTS: 1
143. ANS: E   PTS: 1
144. ANS: H   PTS: 1
145. ANS: M   PTS: 1
146. ANS: B   PTS: 1
147. ANS: K   PTS: 1
148. ANS: J   PTS: 1
149. ANS: L   PTS: 1
150. ANS: G   PTS: 1
151. ANS: A   PTS: 1
152. ANS: F   PTS: 1

153. ANS: H   PTS: 1
154. ANS: G   PTS: 1
155. ANS: K   PTS: 1

156. ANS: M   PTS: 1
157. ANS: I   PTS: 1
158. ANS: J   PTS: 1
159. ANS: C   PTS: 1
160. ANS: D   PTS: 1
161. ANS: B   PTS: 1

162. ANS: D   PTS: 1
163. ANS: E   PTS: 1
164. ANS: F   PTS: 1
165. ANS: H   PTS: 1
166. ANS: A   PTS: 1
167. ANS: G   PTS: 1
168. ANS: B   PTS: 1
169. ANS: C   PTS: 1
170. ANS: J   PTS: 1

171. ANS: G   PTS: 1
172. ANS: D   PTS: 1
173. ANS: I   PTS: 1
174. ANS: A   PTS: 1
175. ANS: F   PTS: 1
176. ANS: J   PTS: 1
177. ANS: H   PTS: 1
178. ANS: C   PTS: 1
179. ANS: E   PTS: 1
180. ANS: B   PTS: 1

COMPLETION

181. ANS: Accreditation

     PTS: 1

182. ANS: denial, anger, bargaining, depression, acceptance (in any order)

     PTS: 1

183. ANS: Hospice

     PTS: 1

184. ANS: positive

     PTS: 1

185. ANS: clinical, administrative

PTS: 1
186. ANS: Professionalism

PTS: 1
187. ANS: professional publications, educational seminars, Internet research, professional organization membership

PTS: 1
188. ANS: recertification

PTS: 1
189. ANS: empathy, service

PTS: 1
190. ANS: service

PTS: 1
191. ANS: terminology

PTS: 1
192. ANS: career

PTS: 1
193. ANS: oral communication

PTS: 1
194. ANS: Medical Assistant's Creed

PTS: 1
195. ANS: negative

PTS: 1
196. ANS: government, nongovernment

PTS: 1
197. ANS: nonprofit

PTS: 1
198. ANS: For-profit

PTS: 1
199. ANS: beds

PTS: 1
200. ANS: staff privileges

PTS: 1
201. ANS: admitting

PTS: 1
202. ANS: nuclear medicine

PTS: 1
203. ANS: patients

PTS: 1
204. ANS: skills

PTS: 1
205. ANS: adjunct

PTS: 1
206. ANS: medical center

PTS: 1
207. ANS: Laboratories

PTS: 1
208. ANS: Specialized care

PTS: 1
209. ANS: diagnosis, treatment

PTS: 1
210. ANS: precision, accuracy

PTS: 1
211. ANS: defendant

PTS: 1
212. ANS: bioethics

PTS: 1
213. ANS: medical conduct, ethics

PTS: 1
214. ANS: Lasagna Professional Oath

PTS: 1
215. ANS: Principles of Medical Ethics

PTS: 1
216. ANS: rebate

PTS: 1
217. ANS: policies

PTS: 1
218. ANS: confidential

PTS: 1
219. ANS: medical etiquette

PTS: 1
220. ANS: supervisor, employer

PTS: 1
221. ANS: quackery

PTS: 1
222. ANS: claims made, claims incurred

PTS: 1
223. ANS: *Respondeat superior*

PTS: 1
224. ANS: grievance committee

PTS: 1
225. ANS: Subpoena duces tecum

PTS: 1
226. ANS: active listening

PTS: 1
227. ANS: face

PTS: 1
228. ANS: Aggression

PTS: 1
229. ANS: barrier

PTS: 1
230. ANS: stereotyping

PTS: 1
231. ANS: noncompliant

PTS: 1
232. ANS: paraphrasing

PTS: 1
233. ANS: open-ended

PTS: 1
234. ANS: neutral

PTS: 1
235. ANS: communication cycle

PTS: 1
236. ANS: hearing

PTS: 1
237. ANS: white-coat syndrome

PTS: 1
238. ANS: attitude

PTS: 1
239. ANS: hierarchy of needs

PTS: 1
240. ANS: rationalization

PTS: 1

SHORT ANSWER

241. ANS:
The administrative medical assistant should focus on finding solutions.

PTS: 1
242. ANS:
An effective health care worker should be skilled at understanding human behavior because people react differently to situations.

PTS: 1
243. ANS:

The patient is trained to take total responsibility for his own or family's health from birth to death and to develop a lifestyle that produces wellness.

PTS: 1

244. ANS:
Yes. The medical assistant will use them repeatedly when employed in the medical field.

PTS: 1

245. ANS:
A Patient's Bill of Rights was developed to try to remedy some recurring complaints about attitudes of and treatment by physicians and administrators. Also, it can help reduce malpractice suits because these often result from misunderstandings between the patient and physician or hospital.

PTS: 1

246. ANS:
Minors are considered emancipated when they are: (a) living apart from their parents or guardians and managing their own financial affairs; (b) married or divorced at any age; (c) on active duty in the military service; (d) college students living away from home even when financially dependent on their parents; (e) becoming a parent (even if not married).

PTS: 1

247. ANS:
Physiologic needs, safety needs, love and belonging needs, esteem needs, self-actualization needs.

PTS: 1

248. ANS:
Any five of the following: (a) apathy, (b) aggression, (c) avoidance, (d) compensation, (e) denial, (f) displacement, (g) projection, (h) rationalization, (i) regression, (j) repression, (k) sarcasm, and (l) undoing.

PTS: 1

249. ANS:
Good communicators focus on others, paying attention to everything the other person is trying to communicate. Good communicators know that what they have said is only the beginning of the communication cycle.

Poor communicators focus on themselves, their own thoughts, feelings, experiences, and ideas. Poor communicators speak their part and think that the communication is over.

PTS: 1

250. ANS:
Answers will include three of the following: (a) repeating, (b) paraphrasing, (c) questioning, (d) requesting examples, (e) summarizing, or (f) the silent pause.

PTS: 1

Exam 2

True/False
Indicate whether the statement is true or false.

_____ 1. Because of right-to-privacy laws, it is now mandatory to protect the patient's privacy.

_____ 2. It should be standard practice to get to know patients' names and to learn how they prefer to be addressed.

_____ 3. Patients should be expected to wait as long as necessary in the reception area.

_____ 4. To retain privacy, the registration form should be destroyed after the patient's first visit is completed.

_____ 5. After greeting the patient, the receptionist should ensure that all registration and insurance information is current and up to date.

_____ 6. It is not the receptionist's responsibility to be familiar with mobility devices used by elderly or physically impaired patients.

_____ 7. To ensure eye contact, it is important to try and speak to a disabled person at eye level.

_____ 8. If the receptionist will be away from the work station, the screen saver should be activated to protect any open documents from unauthorized viewing.

_____ 9. Toys with small parts should be available to entertain children of all ages in the waiting area.

_____ 10. Telephone guidelines include using expression in your tone.

_____ 11. The assistant should cultivate a cheerful and excited voice, speaking with inflections at the end of sentences.

_____ 12. The manner in which the assistant speaks will determine the caller's response.

_____ 13. Cellular signals are secure.

_____ 14. Once you purchase a cellular phone, you may use it with no charge at any time.

_____ 15. Basic etiquette requires that the return call of a pager message be made at a quiet, private location.

_____ 16. If a caller refuses to identify herself, you should connect her to the doctor immediately.

_____ 17. Follow-up examinations require 45- to 60-minute appointments, whereas patients seen for the first time at fixed intervals are usually assigned between 15 and 30 minutes.

_____ 18. Appointment time allotments will vary depending on the physicians' specialty and the circumstances.

_____ 19. To improve scheduling, only one emergency slot should be scheduled during the day.

_____ 20. Postoperative visits are made at the hospital by the physician at least once or twice daily.

_____ 21. In a group practice, colleagues may alternate hospital rounds.

_____ 22. House calls are made more frequently today because physicians can treat fewer patients in more time in their offices.

_____ 23. In order to determine if the appointment schedule is adequate for the needs of the patients and the office, schedule tracking should be done for 6-12 weeks.

_____ 24. In a phonetic filing system, letters in a lengthy surname after the 3-digit code has been determined would be ignored.

_____ 25. Medical and financial records should be filed together.

_____ 26. General filing rules should be written so all staff members are following the same guidelines.

_____ 27. No two subject files would be the same.

_____ 28. If two names are identical, the address may be used to make the filing decision.

_____ 29. Most physicians discard patient files after three to five years of inactivity.

_____ 30. Micrographics are small pictures placed on the outside of folders that serve as alerts.

Multiple Choice
Identify the choice that best completes the statement or answers the question.

_____ 31. Before the patient arrives, the assistant should
   a. watch for the patient's arrival and be able to greet him by name.
   b. allow the patient privacy by not greeting him.
   c. take no extra measures to greet the patient so that all patients are treated equally.
   d. read all of the entries in the patient's chart to become familiar with his case.

_____ 32. Use of a patient sign-in sheet is
   a. encouraged so that patients can get to know each others' names.
   b. legally a breach of confidentiality if it allows patients to view the names of all previous patients seen that day.
   c. discouraged because it increases the chance of a waiting patient's being overlooked.
   d. not considered a violation of privacy.

_____ 33. A personalized greeting
   a. conveys an unprofessional environment.
   b. builds trust and confidence.
   c. should never involve touching the patient.
   d. should always include calling the patient by his first name.

_____ 34. Which of the following is NOT an appropriate <u>welcoming</u> remark?
   a. Good morning, Mrs. Jones.
   b. Hello, Mr. Smith.
   c. Nice to see you, Ms. Hall.
   d. Hello, John. How are you?

_____ 35. When patients have spent more than 30 minutes in the waiting room,
   a. they should be told to keep waiting.
   b. they should be given an option to reschedule.
   c. tell them it will just be a few more minutes
   d. do nothing because patients generally expect to wait 60 minutes or longer.

_____ 36. Individuals who are physically impaired

a. should be scheduled allowing extra appointment time.
b. may need parking closer to the door.
c. may need assistance getting into the office.
d. all of the above.

_____ 37. Managed care insurance plans
a. may need preauthorization for some services.
b. always cover preventive health services.
c. always cover vision examinations.
d. all of the above.

_____ 38. A medical history form
a. is only completed by returning patients.
b. is sent to the patient's former physician to gather information.
c. should be completed by each new patient.
d. is never completed by an established patient.

_____ 39. A patient instruction form may include
a. medications.
b. precautions.
c. date of next appointment.
d. all of the above.

_____ 40. The reception area
a. should always be kept clean and neat.
b. should include a smoking area.
c. should be kept cold to keep costs down.
d. should always have beautiful, fresh flowers.

_____ 41. If the office is orderly, the surroundings clean and cheerful, and the receptionist friendly and well-groomed, patients will be
a. clean and cheerful.
b. friendly.
c. more relaxed.
d. happy.

_____ 42. Toys for children in the reception area should
a. consist of many small parts.
b. be easily broken.
c. produce a variety of sounds or noises.
d. none of the above.

_____ 43. The ideal thermostat setting for the reception room is
a. 64 to 66 degrees.
b. 68 to 70 degrees.
c. 74 to 76 degrees.
d. 76 to 78 degrees.

_____ 44. Which of the following is an important safety feature of the waiting area?
a. The carpet should be in good repair.
b. Unused electrical outlets should have safety covers.
c. Electrical cords should be placed behind furniture.
d. All of the above.

_____ 45. Which of the following is inappropriate in a patient waiting room?
a. Magazines
b. Fragrant flowers
c. Water cooler
d. Educational brochures

_____ 46. If a patient refuses to divulge information on the registration form,
a. the patient may be expected to pay at the time of service.
b. it is okay, the information is all optional anyway.

c. refuse service to the patient.

d. the office personnel do not have to be polite to that patient.

_____ 47. The first thing a receptionist should do when a patient enters the office is

a. request the insurance information.   c. close all computer applications.

b. greet the patient.   d. escort the patient to an exam room.

_____ 48. Before the patient leaves the office, the receptionist should

a. obtain a copy of the patient's insurance card.

b. have the patient complete the registration form.

c. give the patient a copy of the privacy notice.

d. make sure a follow-up visit, if indicated, has been scheduled.

_____ 49. The process of determining what type of incoming telephone call is being received and deciding which person should receive the call is known as

a. screening.   c. telecommunication.

b. telephone triage.   d. protocol

_____ 50. Placing, receiving, and screening telephone calls is a responsibility for the medical assistant; it would be considered

a. a routine task.   c. important for public relations.

b. part of billing and collection duties.   d. triage.

_____ 51. Which of the following telephone guidelines is accurate?

a. Be very relaxed and familiar with the caller.

b. Let your voice imply that the caller is interrupting you so you do not waste valuable time.

c. Repeat the caller's name during the conversation to show attentiveness.

d. Never smile while you are on the phone.

_____ 52. A wireless telephone that communicates through antenna towers is known as a/an

a. answering service.   c. speakerphone.

b. cellular telephone.   d. voice mail system.

_____ 53. When taking a phone message from a patient, you should be sure to record

a. the date and time.   c. the reason for the call.

b. the patient's name and phone number.   d. all of the above.

_____ 54. Which piece of telephone equipment reduces phone fatigue and allows mobility?

a. Wireless headset   c. Cellular phone

b. Touch-tone phone   d. Answering service

_____ 55. You may experience interference when using what type of telephone in mountainous or airport areas?

a. Electronic telephone   c. Cellular telephone

b. Speaker telephone   d. Automated attendant telephone

_____ 56. Which of the following guidelines regarding voice mail is accurate?

a. Keep the message short.

b. Do not commit yourself to when you will be returning the call.

c. Instruct the caller to leave a message in the event of an emergency.

d. Tell the caller to call back during office hours.

_____ 57. A business that specializes in taking and relaying telephone messages when offices are closed is a/an

a. automated attendant.   c. voice pager system.

b. cellular telephone.   d. answering service.

58. When using an automated attendant answering system, there should always be an option that allows the caller to
    a. talk to the physician directly.
    b. talk to a live person.
    c. access the complicated triage system.
    d. page the physician.

59. Triage means to
    a. interrupt the physician if she is with a patient already.
    b. put the caller on hold and ask advice from the physician.
    c. sort things out.
    d. consider three options before making any decisions.

60. A telephone log is important
    a. because it provides a permanent chronological record.
    b. for medicolegal reasons.
    c. both a and b.
    d. neither a nor b.

61. Reference instructions that need to be followed in determining how to triage a telephone call are referred to as
    a. competencies.
    b. protocols.
    c. documents.
    d. policies.

62. When a caller will not terminate a conversation, it is appropriate to say
    a. "Unfortunately, I can't stay on the phone with you all day."
    b. "I have to go now" (and hang up quickly before anything else is said).
    c. "Let me see if I understand what you are saying."
    d. "I am sorry, Mrs. Snyder, but I need to assist another patient right now."

63. According to studies, which of the following makes two-thirds of telephone callers angry?
    a. Having to repeat themselves
    b. Leaving a message
    c. Being put on hold
    d. Talking slowly

64. Whether it is an incoming or outgoing call, be sure the party you are speaking with is properly
    a. identified
    b. authorized
    c. interrogated
    d. managed

65. If the physician receives a personal call from a family member, the medical assistant should
    a. only take a message.
    b. ask nursing staff to take a message.
    c. connect the caller to the physician.
    d. tell the family member to call back.

66. An incoming telephone call should be answered before the
    a. first ring.
    b. second ring.
    c. third ring.
    d. fifth ring.

67. The appointment abbreviation "stat" stands for
    a. immediately.
    b. emergency.
    c. diagnosis.
    d. none of the above.

68. The appointment abbreviation "DX" stands for
    a. did not keep appointment.
    b. diagnosis.
    c. dressing change.
    d. discontinue.

69. More patients complain about
    a. the temperature in the waiting room than about waiting time.
    b. high fees than about waiting time.
    c. co-payments and deductibles than anything else.

d. waiting time than about high fees.

70. How should sales people or drug detail representatives' visits be handled?
    a. Do not schedule appointments for them as they tend to annoy the physician.
    b. Block out one day per month for sales/detail representatives.
    c. Block off one or two quiet periods in the middle of the week for sales/detail representatives.
    d. Make sure to block off a lot of time for these because they may bring drug samples.

71. Which of the following is the best way for the medical assistant to handle a true emergency situation?
    a. Diagnose the situation and prescribe treatment over the phone.
    b. Refer the patient to a hospital emergency facility.
    c. Schedule the patient to come in at the end of the workday when all other patients have been seen.
    d. Refer the call to someone else.

72. The scheduling technique that allows patients to walk in during a specified time frame and be seen in the order they arrive is
    a. stream scheduling.   c. double booking.
    b. triage scheduling.   d. open hours.

73. Which type of scheduling works well when the staff knows how to get relevant information from the patient so a real emergency can be handled promptly?
    a. Stream scheduling   c. Double booking
    b. Triage scheduling   d. Clustering

74. Which type of scheduling works well for specialty and consulting practices because it allows the physician time to prepare for each office visit with the knowledge that the day will begin and end on schedule if patients adhere to their assigned times?
    a. Stream scheduling   c. Double booking
    b. Triage scheduling   d. Open hours scheduling

75. In what type of scheduling system are patients told that their appointments are on the hour and each is seen in the order in which they arrive?
    a. True wave   c. Clustering
    b. Modified wave   d. Single booking

76. Which type of scheduling method allows patients to schedule appointments on the same day they call?
    a. True wave   c. Clustered appointment
    b. Open access   d. Modified wave

77. When setting up preoperative appointments and tests for a patient,
    a. schedule all tests and procedures as close together as possible.
    b. remember that an ill patient may find too many appointments in one tiring.
    c. schedule them as far apart as possible.
    d. only take into consideration when the physician wants them done.

78. To avoid an audit and improve scheduling,
    a. track all waiting times.
    b. notify patients if the physician is off schedule.
    c. notify the supervisor immediately when a patient with an urgent complaint cannot

be given an appointment on the same day.

d. all of the above.

79. All appointment cancellations or no-shows should
    a. be disregarded.
    b. be rescheduled immediately.
    c. be documented in the patient's chart.
    d. result in immediate discharge of the patient.

80. A printout showing all of the appointments scheduled for the day is called a/an
    a. appointment reference sheet.   c. auditing sheet.
    b. personal organizer.   d. appointment reminder card.

81. What is the name of a pressboard sheet used to direct the eye to a section of file and to provide support for records?
    a. Guide   c. Label
    b. Cut   d. Shelf

82. A sticker to attach to the tab or other part of a folder is called the
    a. guide.   c. label.
    b. cut.   d. alert.

83. Creases along the lower front flap of a folder to allow for expansion by folding each crease are known as
    a. micrographics.   c. cuts.
    b. scores.   d. tabs.

84. What is placed in the file cabinet or substituted for a file when it is removed from a file drawer?
    a. Tickler   c. Master patient index
    b. Micrograph   d. Outguide

85. Filmed records reduced in size to save space are referred to as
    a. tickler files.   c. outguides.
    b. micrographics.   d. scanners.

86. What is the name for a type of follow-up file?
    a. Tickler   c. Outguide
    b. Micrograph   d. Index

87. What is the simplest and most popular filing method that is easy to understand and does not require a cross-reference index?
    a. Alphabetic name sequence   c. Phonetic filing
    b. Numeric filing   d. Dates

88. What type of filing system might be preferable if privacy and convenience of expansion are important considerations?
    a. Chronologic   c. Phonetic
    b. Indirect   d. Alphabetic

89. In what filing system would names like Smythe and Smith be filed together?
    a. Alphabetic   c. Phonetic
    b. Numeric   d. Indexing

90. Approximately how many records will an open-shelf file unit with seven 36-inch shelves hold?
    a. 250   c. 750
    b. 500   d. 1,000

91. Which type of file cabinets are popular in medical offices because they require less floor space than other types?
   a. Open-shelf lateral files
   b. Vertical cabinets
   c. Conventional steel drawers
   d. Automated files

92. The size of the tab on the back of a folder is known as the
   a. guide.
   b. cut.
   c. label.
   d. score.

93. In alphabetic filing, names are divided into sections called
   a. surname.
   b. units.
   c. codes.
   d. tabs.

94. There is an alphabetic filing rule which states "file
   a. something before nothing."
   b. anything before something."
   c. nothing before something."
   d. anything before nothing."

95. Which indexing unit is the last name according to alphabetic filing rules?
   a. First
   b. Second
   c. Third
   d. Fourth

96. When searching for a missing patient folder,
   a. check in front of and behind where the folder should be.
   b. look to see if the folder was filed under the patient's first name.
   c. search the entire section of the first letter of the patient's last name.
   d. all of the above.

97. What should be done periodically to protect computerized files in case there is a power surge, computer breakdown, or virus?
   a. Purge
   b. Recycle
   c. Scan
   d. Backup

98. According to the alphabetic filing rules, which of the following names would come before Smith?
   a. Smythe
   b. Smithson
   c. Smieth
   d. Smithe

99. According to the alphabetic filing rules, which of the following names would be after Thompson?
   a. Thomson
   b. Thomas
   c. Thomason
   d. Thommpson

100. According to the alphabetic rules of filing, which name would be filed first?
   a. A. C. Albertson
   b. A. C. Alberts
   c. C. A. Albert
   d. Al Berts

Matching

Match each term with the correct statement below.
   a. biohazard
   b. face sheet
   c. hazardous waste
   d. infectious waste
   e. patient instruction form
   f. patient/practice information brochure
   g. professionalism
   h. reception room
   i. registration form
   j. universal precautions

_____ 101. treat all waste as if it were infectious

_____102. an outer office provided for patients who are awaiting appointments
_____103. form given to the patient at the end of a visit that outlines the doctor's instructions and treatment plan
_____104. includes blood, urine, or human waste
_____105. printed material explaining office policies and procedures
_____106. substance that poses a threat to human health
_____107. document with hospital admission information
_____108. a fill-in sheet, completed by all patients prior to their initial visit
_____109. conduct, aims, and qualities characteristic of a skilled medical assistant

Match each term with the correct statement below.

a. answering machine	j. speakerphone
b. answering service	k. telecommunication
c. callback	l. telephone decision grid
d. cellular telephone	m. telephone log
e. conference call	n. telephone reference aid
f. emergency care	o. toll call
g. pager	p. triage
h. protocol	q. urgent care
i. screening	r. voice mail

_____110. stores and forwards messages, combines elements of the telephone and computer, and has a recording device which permits one-way messages
_____111. process of evaluating to determine the action to be taken on a telephone call
_____112. telephone call linking several persons at different geographical locations in one conversation
_____113. record of types of incoming calls identifying the action to be taken
_____114. alphabetic list of frequently called telephone numbers
_____115. telephone call within a large metropolitan area charged at a unit rate
_____116. protocol for allocation of patients for treatment by order of urgency and importance
_____117. transmission of voice and/or data over a wire/line
_____118. written, dated record of all telephone calls, also noting the action taken
_____119. telephone with a microphone designed for hands-free communication
_____120. set of instructions used for reference prescribing strict adherence to correct etiquette
_____121. term indicating that a return telephone call is necessary
_____122. treatment of a condition that needs attention within 24 hours
_____123. wireless telephone that communicates through antenna towers
_____124. immediate treatment when a person's life is in danger
_____125. A business that handles telephone calls when the office is closed
_____126. handheld, one-way communication device

Match each term with the correct statement below.

a. appointment abbreviations	i. new patient
b. appointment book	j. no-show
c. appointment card	k. open access
d. appointment schedule	l. PDA

e. clustering   m. referral
f. established patient   n. software
g. fixed interval   o. template
h. modified wave   p. true wave

_____127. handheld computer

_____128. patient who has not received services in the past three years from any physician of the same specialty in a group practice

_____129. system of advance appointment scheduling in which patients are allocated specific periods of time for their office visits

_____130. patient who does not keep a scheduled appointment and does not call the office to cancel

_____131. procedure followed when a primary care physician recommends another physician for further medical treatment

_____132. act of scheduling patients with similar ailments in group sequence

_____133. guide for scheduling various types of appointments

_____134. patient who has received services within the past three years from any physician of the same specialty in a group practice

_____135. set of sheets used to schedule patients' time in the office

_____136. list designating fixed times for patient appointments

_____137. small card showing the day, date, and time of an appointment and given to a patient to serve as a reminder

_____138. same-day scheduling

_____139. appointments are scheduled on the hour and patients are seen in the order they arrive

_____140. instructions that direct the computer to perform a task

Match each term with the correct statement below.
a. alphabetic filing   f. diagnostic file
b. backup   g. encryption
c. topic   h. given name
d. charge-out system   i. indexing unit
e. chronological filing   j. master patient index

_____141. in subject filing, a name under which records are filed

_____142. a procedure for accounting for items removed from files

_____143. exact copy of data on the hard drive

_____144. information learned from patient case histories and filed for reference

_____145. file by date

_____146. an individual's first name

_____147. listing of numbers assigned to each patient's file

_____148. files organized by letters of the alphabet

_____149. in filing, the order in which parts of a name are considered

_____150. files are stored in coded form

Match each term with the correct statement below.
a. micrographics   f. purge

b. numeric filing
c. lateral file cabinets
d. outguide
e. phonetic filing

g. recycle
h. subject filing
i. surname
j. tickler

____151. information is reduced on film to save storage space
____152. file cabinets with shelves for record storage
____153. an individual's last name
____154. processing waste for reuse
____155. an arrangement of records in number sequence
____156. procedure to remove outdated items from file folders or computer disks
____157. filing by sound, rather than letter
____158. used as a reminder or follow-up file
____159. alphabetic arrangement of files by topic or theme
____160. substitution card placed when a file has been removed

Completion
Complete each statement.

161. The _____ _____ is where patients wait until the physician is ready to see them.

162. When arriving at the office in the morning, the receptionist should retrieve all phone messages from the _____ _____.

163. Legally, a sign-in sheet where all patients can view each others' signatures can be a breach of _____.

164. As the first one to greet the patient, the receptionist sets the tone for the visit with a/an _____, a helpful _____, and a caring _____.

165. Medical records for _____ _____ are usually pulled and prepared the evening before the appointment date.

166. Charts for _____ _____ are made up either the evening before the appointment or the morning of the appointment.

167. A comprehensive and concise _____ _____, designed to index a patient's personal data and insurance information, should be completed on or before a patient's first office visit.

168. When speaking to a patient, customize comments by adding the _____ _____ to prevent you from sounding like a broken record.

169. A/An _____ _____ hung in the reception room can be filled with interesting items for patients to look at.

170. The medical assistant who establishes positive personal relations will build _____ and _____.

171. If the receptionist is on the phone when a patient arrives in the office, the receptionist should still _____ the arrival of the patient with a smile or a nod.

172. After the patient is registered, a/an _____ _____ must be given to and signed by the patient.

173. A sign in the waiting room should read "Please approach the reception desk if you have waited more than _____."

174. Patients who are _____ _____ may have deformities that alter their functions or appearance.

175. When speaking to a physically impaired person, try to position yourself at eye level with the patient so that you can ensure _____ _____.

176. The application for disabled person parking plates will need to be signed by the _____.

177. Use _____ _____, treating all waste as if it were infectious.

178. A/An _____ container should be available for disposal of hazardous and/or infectious wastes.

179. If a patient should stop breathing in the reception room, and the physician is not immediately available, the receptionist should be prepared to start _____ _____.

180. In order to give clear directions, the medical assistant must have good _____ skills.

181. Another term used for conference calls is _____.

182. It has been said that telephone techniques can mean the _____ or _____ of a medical practice.

183. A multiphysician clinic in a city would need more _____ _____ than a one-doctor office in a rural location.

184. To improve telephone techniques, use the words "_____" and "_____ _____" frequently.

185. Direct any call of a clinical nature to a clinical medical assistant who can then route the call to the appropriate _____.

186. _____ _____ is a special telephone feature that will automatically redirect incoming telephone calls.

187. _____ signals are not secure.

188. _____ _____ is a type of answering system that combines the technology of a telephone, a computer, and a recording device.

189. A/An _____ _____ situation is one in which a person's life is in danger.

190. The use of a/an _____ _____ is not recommended in the medical office because an anxious caller needs comforting through personal contact.

191. When placing a/an _____ call for the physician, the medical assistant assembles patient data before initiating the call, dials direct, and keeps the conversation brief.

192. When placing calls within a large city or out of state, the medical assistant should make use of _____ numbers whenever possible.

193. When managing a/an _____ call, it is important to remain calm and verify all information with the caller.

194. When a patient calls requesting a/an _____ _____, it is important to get the name and phone number of the pharmacy the patient uses.

195. A patient might be on a/an _____ list because she is trying a new medication.

196. _____ visits are appointments after surgery.

197. When a patient is habitually late for appointments, they should be scheduled for _____ minutes before the real appointment time.

198. Several _____ slots should be available on the daily schedule.

199. The four basic considerations that should determine the scheduling of all appointments are the _____ of the patient, the scheduling _____ and habits of the physician, and availability of medical _____ and _____.

200. A patient's need for a/an _____ appointment will be decided by the physician and the patient at the close of a visit.

201. Poor appointment scheduling may provide an excuse for a Managed Care Organization to closely _____ a practice's patient relations and medical outcomes.

202. If quality of care has suffered due to poor appointment scheduling, a Managed Care Organization may drop the practice from its _____ of physicians.

203. The _____ _____ card is sent to the patient before the appointment and will greatly reduce the chance of the patient being a no-show.

204. _____ _____ are shortened terms used to indicate the reason that the patient is coming in.

205. Waiting times of _____ or longer sharply reduce the likelihood that men would visit a doctor again.

206. A/An _____ _____ _____ is a handheld computer that can serve as an organizer or note taker when the physician sees patients outside of the office.

207. A computer _____ program is used for appointment scheduling in most offices.

208. The medical assistant makes preoperative appointments for _____ _____ and may also schedule appointments for their _____ _____, and _____.

209. Notify patients if the physician is running _____ minutes or more behind schedule.

210. The _____ _____ _____ should always be part of the surgical planning process to make sure that all sequential tasks are completed.

211. In _____ _____ scheduling, patients are scheduled for the first half of each hour, and the second half of each hour is left for walk-in, work-in, or emergency patients.

212. _____ _____ scheduling allows patients to walk in anytime within a specific time frame, and they are seen in order of their arrival.

213. It is important to _____ all appointments the moment they are made.

214. Some examples of _____ testing are laboratory tests, x-rays, an EKG, or a bone scan.

215. When scheduling a surgical procedure, the medical assistant should call the hospital _____ department to make arrangements for the patient to enter the hospital and stay after the surgery.

216. The simplest and most popular filing method is the _____ filing system.

217. A collection of information stored electronically is referred to as a/an _____.

218. _____ filing is the alphabetic arrangement of records by topic.

219. In a hospital or large facility indirect filing system, _____ _____ is used when file expansion is not necessary because a patient receives a new number and folder at each visit.

220. In a/an _____ filing system, _____ letters are used rather than 26.

221. _____ files should always be backed up at the end of the _____.

222. A process known as _____ makes data look like gibberish to unauthorized users.

223. When filing subjects, one way to avoid misfiling is to keep the _____ as simple as possible.

224. A/an _____ is a substitution card which will be put in the place of a folder that has been removed.

225. In 1986, the Association of Records Managers and Administrators Inc. developed the rules for _____ that are the basis for most alphabetic filing systems in use today.

226. _____ _____ is used in addition to alphabetic filing or numeric filing as an added visual cue to assist in filing.

227. _____ are designed to hold information to be stored in lateral file cabinets' vertical file drawers.

228. Because the security of medical records is important, it is essential that filing cabinets have a/an _____ mechanism.

229. When names are identical, _____ are then used as the next indexing unit.

230. _____ files usually found in large hospital facilities bring the records to the individual operator for retrieval.

Short Answer

231. What should be the intent of the printed patient/practice information brochure?

232. List five items that might be included on a patient instruction form.

233. How should you end a telephone call?

234. Explain five things the assistant should do when receiving a complaint from an angry caller.

235. Describe how to determine if a scheduling system is satisfying patient needs and is flexible enough for the practice.

236. Is it advisable to schedule a patient appointment more than one month in advance? Why or why not?

237. Describe the difference between a new patient and an established patient.

238. Describe the first three steps the medical assistant should take if a record cannot be found.

239. List three office management considerations used when determining a filing system.

240. List the indexing units of the following: Jefferson Community Health Center.

Exam 2
Answer Section

TRUE/FALSE

    1. ANS: T   PTS: 1
    2. ANS: T   PTS: 1
    3. ANS: F   PTS: 1
    4. ANS: F   PTS: 1
    5. ANS: T   PTS: 1
    6. ANS: F   PTS: 1
    7. ANS: T   PTS: 1
    8. ANS: T   PTS: 1
    9. ANS: F   PTS: 1
  10. ANS: T   PTS: 1
  11. ANS: F   PTS: 1
  12. ANS: T   PTS: 1
  13. ANS: F   PTS: 1
  14. ANS: F   PTS: 1
  15. ANS: T   PTS: 1
  16. ANS: F   PTS: 1
  17. ANS: F   PTS: 1
  18. ANS: T   PTS: 1
  19. ANS: F   PTS: 1
  20. ANS: T   PTS: 1
  21. ANS: T   PTS: 1
  22. ANS: F   PTS: 1
  23. ANS: T   PTS: 1
  24. ANS: T   PTS: 1
  25. ANS: F   PTS: 1
  26. ANS: T   PTS: 1
  27. ANS: T   PTS: 1
  28. ANS: T   PTS: 1
  29. ANS: F   PTS: 1
  30. ANS: F   PTS: 1

MULTIPLE CHOICE

  31. ANS: A   PTS: 1
  32. ANS: B   PTS: 1
  33. ANS: B   PTS: 1
  34. ANS: D   PTS: 1

35. ANS: B	PTS: 1
36. ANS: D	PTS: 1
37. ANS: A	PTS: 1
38. ANS: C	PTS: 1
39. ANS: D	PTS: 1
40. ANS: A	PTS: 1
41. ANS: C	PTS: 1
42. ANS: D	PTS: 1
43. ANS: B	PTS: 1
44. ANS: D	PTS: 1
45. ANS: B	PTS: 1
46. ANS: A	PTS: 1
47. ANS: B	PTS: 1
48. ANS: D	PTS: 1
49. ANS: A	PTS: 1
50. ANS: C	PTS: 1
51. ANS: C	PTS: 1
52. ANS: B	PTS: 1
53. ANS: D	PTS: 1
54. ANS: A	PTS: 1
55. ANS: C	PTS: 1
56. ANS: A	PTS: 1
57. ANS: D	PTS: 1
58. ANS: B	PTS: 1
59. ANS: C	PTS: 1
60. ANS: C	PTS: 1
61. ANS: B	PTS: 1
62. ANS: D	PTS: 1
63. ANS: C	PTS: 1
64. ANS: A	PTS: 1
65. ANS: C	PTS: 1
66. ANS: C	PTS: 1
67. ANS: A	PTS: 1
68. ANS: B	PTS: 1
69. ANS: D	PTS: 1
70. ANS: C	PTS: 1
71. ANS: B	PTS: 1
72. ANS: D	PTS: 1
73. ANS: B	PTS: 1
74. ANS: A	PTS: 1
75. ANS: A	PTS: 1
76. ANS: B	PTS: 1
77. ANS: B	PTS: 1

78.	ANS: D	PTS: 1
79.	ANS: C	PTS: 1
80.	ANS: A	PTS: 1
81.	ANS: A	PTS: 1
82.	ANS: C	PTS: 1
83.	ANS: B	PTS: 1
84.	ANS: D	PTS: 1
85.	ANS: B	PTS: 1
86.	ANS: A	PTS: 1
87.	ANS: A	PTS: 1
88.	ANS: B	PTS: 1
89.	ANS: C	PTS: 1
90.	ANS: D	PTS: 1
91.	ANS: A	PTS: 1
92.	ANS: B	PTS: 1
93.	ANS: B	PTS: 1
94.	ANS: C	PTS: 1
95.	ANS: A	PTS: 1
96.	ANS: D	PTS: 1
97.	ANS: D	PTS: 1
98.	ANS: C	PTS: 1
99.	ANS: A	PTS: 1
100.	ANS: C	PTS: 1

MATCHING

101.	ANS: J	PTS: 1
102.	ANS: H	PTS: 1
103.	ANS: E	PTS: 1
104.	ANS: D	PTS: 1
105.	ANS: F	PTS: 1
106.	ANS: A	PTS: 1
107.	ANS: B	PTS: 1
108.	ANS: I	PTS: 1
109.	ANS: G	PTS: 1
110.	ANS: R	PTS: 1
111.	ANS: I	PTS: 1
112.	ANS: E	PTS: 1
113.	ANS: L	PTS: 1
114.	ANS: N	PTS: 1
115.	ANS: O	PTS: 1
116.	ANS: P	PTS: 1

117.	ANS: K	PTS: 1
118.	ANS: M	PTS: 1
119.	ANS: J	PTS: 1
120.	ANS: H	PTS: 1
121.	ANS: C	PTS: 1
122.	ANS: Q	PTS: 1
123.	ANS: D	PTS: 1
124.	ANS: F	PTS: 1
125.	ANS: B	PTS: 1
126.	ANS: G	PTS: 1

127.	ANS: L	PTS: 1
128.	ANS: I	PTS: 1
129.	ANS: G	PTS: 1
130.	ANS: J	PTS: 1
131.	ANS: M	PTS: 1
132.	ANS: E	PTS: 1
133.	ANS: O	PTS: 1
134.	ANS: F	PTS: 1
135.	ANS: B	PTS: 1
136.	ANS: D	PTS: 1
137.	ANS: C	PTS: 1
138.	ANS: K	PTS: 1
139.	ANS: P	PTS: 1
140.	ANS: N	PTS: 1

141.	ANS: C	PTS: 1
142.	ANS: D	PTS: 1
143.	ANS: B	PTS: 1
144.	ANS: F	PTS: 1
145.	ANS: E	PTS: 1
146.	ANS: H	PTS: 1
147.	ANS: J	PTS: 1
148.	ANS: A	PTS: 1
149.	ANS: I	PTS: 1
150.	ANS: G	PTS: 1

151.	ANS: A	PTS: 1
152.	ANS: C	PTS: 1
153.	ANS: I	PTS: 1
154.	ANS: G	PTS: 1
155.	ANS: B	PTS: 1
156.	ANS: F	PTS: 1

157. ANS: E   PTS: 1
158. ANS: J   PTS: 1
159. ANS: H   PTS: 1
160. ANS: D   PTS: 1

COMPLETION

161. ANS:
reception room
reception area

PTS: 1
162. ANS:
answering service
answering machine

PTS: 1
163. ANS: confidentiality

PTS: 1
164. ANS: smile, attitude, approach

PTS: 1
165. ANS: established patients

PTS: 1
166. ANS: new patients

PTS: 1
167. ANS: registration form

PTS: 1
168. ANS: patient's name

PTS: 1
169. ANS: bulletin board

PTS: 1
170. ANS: trust, confidence

PTS: 1
171. ANS: acknowledge

PTS: 1
172. ANS: privacy notice

PTS: 1
173. ANS: 15 minutes

PTS: 1
174. ANS: physically impaired

PTS: 1
175. ANS: eye contact

PTS: 1
176. ANS: physician

PTS: 1
177. ANS: universal precautions

PTS: 1
178. ANS: biohazard

PTS: 1
179. ANS:
Cardiopulmonary resuscitation
CPR

PTS: 1
180. ANS: communication

PTS: 1
181. ANS: teleconferencing

PTS: 1
182. ANS: success, failure

PTS: 1
183. ANS: telephone lines

PTS: 1
184. ANS: please, thank you

PTS: 1
185. ANS: physician

PTS: 1
186. ANS: Call forwarding

PTS: 1

187. ANS: Cellular

PTS: 1

188. ANS: Voice mail

PTS: 1

189. ANS: emergency care

PTS: 1

190. ANS: answering machine

PTS: 1

191. ANS: long-distance

PTS: 1

192. ANS: toll-free

PTS: 1

193. ANS: emergency

PTS: 1

194. ANS: prescription refill

PTS: 1

195. ANS: callback

PTS: 1

196. ANS: Postoperative

PTS: 1

197. ANS:
15
fifteen

PTS: 1

198. ANS:
emergency
time
appointment

PTS: 1

199. ANS:
needs/convenience/preference
preferences

equipment, facilities/treatment rooms

PTS: 1
200. ANS:
follow-up
return

PTS: 1
201. ANS: monitor

PTS: 1
202. ANS: network

PTS: 1
203. ANS: appointment reminder

PTS: 1
204. ANS: Appointment abbreviations

PTS: 1
205. ANS: 30 minutes

PTS: 1
206. ANS:
Personal Digital Assistant
PDA

PTS: 1
207. ANS: software

PTS: 1
208. ANS: surgical patients, laboratory tests (work), x-rays

PTS: 1
209. ANS:
20
twenty

PTS: 1
210. ANS: surgery flow sheet

PTS: 1
211. ANS: modified wave

PTS: 1

212. ANS: Open hours

    PTS: 1
213. ANS:
    record
    write down

    PTS: 1
214. ANS: diagnostic

    PTS: 1
215. ANS: admissions

    PTS: 1
216. ANS: alphabetic

    PTS: 1
217. ANS: database

    PTS: 1
218. ANS: Subject

    PTS: 1
219. ANS: serial numbering

    PTS: 1
220. ANS:
    phonetic, 6
    phonetic, six

    PTS: 1
221. ANS: Computer, day

    PTS: 1
222. ANS: encryption

    PTS: 1
223. ANS: headings

    PTS: 1
224. ANS: outguide

    PTS: 1
225. ANS: alphabetizing

PTS: 1
226. ANS: Color coding

PTS: 1
227. ANS: Folders

PTS: 1
228. ANS: locking

PTS: 1
229. ANS: addresses

PTS: 1
230. ANS: Automated

PTS: 1

SHORT ANSWER

231. ANS:
The brochure is intended to provide the answers to patients' most commonly asked questions, to act as an effective instrument of communication with patients, and to prevent relationships from deteriorating to the termination point. It reduces telephone calls later on by introducing the physician and the specialty and presenting an image of a practice that is professional in every aspect. Rapport may improve, and the brochure may serve as an effective marketing tool when patients share it with friends and relatives.

PTS: 1
232. ANS:
Any five of the following: (a) patient's name and date of appointment; (b) diagnosis; (c) activities to decrease; (d) activities to increase; (e) medications; (f) precautions; (g) expectations; (h) date of next appointment; (i) signatures of physician and patient to acknowledge patient has been informed.

PTS: 1
233. ANS:
By asking if there are any other questions and thanking the caller, using her name.

PTS: 1
234. ANS:

Any five of the following answers: (a) Identify the person's anger and treat it seriously. (b) Slow down your rate of speech and lower your voice pitch and volume. (c) Remain calm and listen carefully. (d) Do not monopolize the conversation. (e) Change your physical position to regain composure. (f) Repeat information to verify you understand the problem. (g) Express your concern to help and then take action. (h) Document the call. (i) Ask the caller to repeat any instruction you have given her. (j) End the call in a cordial manner. (k) Report the call to the physician or office manager.

PTS: 1

235. ANS:

The staff, including the physician, should periodically review patient flow by analyzing the scheduling for a specific length of time--perhaps one or two weeks--and then adjust the times for required office procedures to better utilize the physician's time and to provide a smoother patient flow.

PTS: 1

236. ANS:

No. It is usually not advisable because the appointment is too easily forgotten.

PTS: 1

237. ANS:

A new patient is one who has never been seen in the office before or who has not been seen by the physician or an associate of the same specialty in a group practice in the past three years. An established patient is one who has been seen within the past three years by the physician or an associate of the same specialty in a group practice.

PTS: 1

238. ANS:

(a) Check in the space just in front of and behind the patient's folder. (b) Check above and below the shelves where the record should be located. (c) Check inside the folders positioned just in front of and behind the one with the missing data.

PTS: 1

239. ANS:

Any three of the following:
amount of active records
amount of inactive records
frequency of record retrieval
amount of filing space
convenience of file locations
cost of the system

PTS: 1

240. ANS:

First indexing unit: Jefferson
Second indexing unit: Community

Third indexing unit: Health
Fourth indexing unit: Center

Exam 3

True/False
Indicate whether the statement is true or false.

_____ 1. Patient records may be used in completing reports on child abuse.

_____ 2. Confidentiality of the medical information must be safeguarded.

_____ 3. Noncontributory, normal, negative, and within normal limits all mean the same thing.

_____ 4. It is a good idea to make up your own set of new abbreviations when you start working in a medical office so that you will be able to create your own system of shorthand.

_____ 5. All medical offices use the same style of record keeping.

_____ 6. Typed entries made during the continuing care of the patient should be signed or initialed by the attending physician.

_____ 7. In hospitals, documents generated via computer may contain electronic signatures.

_____ 8. For industrial/work-related injuries, initial medical reports and progress reports may need to be submitted.

_____ 9. The integrated record system uses flow sheets for tracking each medical problem.

_____ 10. Burns are documented by including the site, size, and number of lesions.

_____ 11. The superscription section of the prescription contains the name of the drug and the quantities of ingredients.

_____ 12. The subscription section of the prescription contains directions to the pharmacist on the total quantity of the drug and the form of the medication.

_____ 13. All prescriptions follow a specific format.

_____ 14. Drug flow sheets may be used to replace the physician's initial dictation in the medical record.

_____ 15. Controlled substances may be flushed down the toilet when they have reached their expiration date.

_____ 16. The Harrison Narcotic Act of 1914 was the beginning of a long history of narcotic control legislation.

_____ 17. All controlled substances have a high potential for abuse and have no medical use.

_____ 18. It is important to document all medication refills in the patient's medical record.

_____ 19. Pharmacists do not provide medication instructions; that is entirely up to the medical office personnel.

_____ 20. The beginning of the memorandum should include who the message is TO, who it is FROM, the DATE, and the SUBJECT.

_____ 21. Ergonomics is the science of developing the most efficient computer software programs.

_____ 22. Electronic typewriters are obsolete and no longer used in any office setting.

_____ 23. There are times when only professionally typed correspondence on business letterhead can convey the desired message and tone.

_____ 24. To make a photocopy, the original material is placed face up on the platen glass.

_____ 25. Any misspelled word makes a letter unmailable.

_____ 26. The modified block letter style has all lines aligned at the left margin.

_____ 27. The inside address on a letter is usually the address of the sender.

_____ 28. Spelling and grammar checks built into word processing software are the only method you should rely on to ensure that correspondence is mailable.

_____ 29. Stamps may be ordered by mail, phone, or online.

_____ 30. With the advent of the Internet, sending First Class letters and other documents using standard mail delivery has increased.

_____ 31. Another name for first-class mail is parcel post.

_____ 32. Occasionally, the medical assistant will need to choose a service endorsement for an envelope to notify the postal service of what is to be done with undeliverable-as-addressed mail or to request an addressee's new address.

_____ 33. Specific typing and addressing standards must be adhered to when preparing an envelope for optical character recognition processing.

_____ 34. To use fax transmission, both the sender and receiver must have a fax machine.

_____ 35. The use of fax transmissions can expedite the diagnostic process, but it is not cost effective.

_____ 36. A window envelope can be used for any address, even if there are six or more lines.

_____ 37. In-office e-mail often serves as a substitute for interoffice memos.

_____ 38. Proper grammar and word usage are not necessary in e-mail communication.

_____ 39. Never forward e-mail chain letters.

_____ 40. A properly completed authorization form is not needed when sending medical records by fax.

Multiple Choice
Identify the choice that best completes the statement or answers the question.

_____ 41. The complexity of medical decision making is based on
   a. the number of diagnoses or management options.
   b. the amount and complexity of data to be reviewed.
   c. the risk of significant complications, morbidity, comorbidities, or mortality.
   d. all of the above.

_____ 42. What would be recorded during an HEENT examination?

a. Shape of the thorax
b. Breath sounds
c. Postnasal drip
d. Patient's mood

43. What would be recorded during a neurologic examination?
a. Heart
b. Cranial nerves
c. Moles
d. Kidneys

44. Laboratory tests
a. may be performed in the office or by an outside laboratory.
b. must be performed by an outside certified laboratory.
c. are interpreted by the medical assistant.
d. none of the above.

45. Evaluation and Management (E/M) services is a phrase used when referring to
a. codes found in the *Current Procedural Terminology* code book.
b. office visits.
c. surgical procedures and management of the patient.
d. both a and b.

46. Usual childhood diseases and previous illnesses are included in the patient's
a. chief complaint.
b. history of present illness.
c. past history.
d. review of systems.

47. Which term describes a part of the examination when the patient's physical characteristics and body parts are observed?
a. Inspection
b. Palpation
c. Percussion
d. Auscultation

48. Which term describes a part of the examination when various parts and organs of the body are touched and felt?
a. Inspection
b. Palpation
c. Percussion
d. Auscultation

49. Temperature, pulse, respiration, and blood pressure are recorded as
a. vital signs.
b. prognosis.
c. diagnosis.
d. chief complaint.

50. When conducting an internal review of medical records, the medical assistant should ensure that
a. all corrections have been made by erasing the incorrect information.
b. there are no handwritten notes in the chart.
c. there is no mention of allergies.
d. there are dates and signatures on every entry in each medical record.

51. SOAP is an acronym for
a. system, observed, auscultation, palpation.
b. subjective, objective, angle, palpation.
c. subjective, objective, assessment, plan.
d. simple, obvious, auscultation, percussion.

52. Which of the following is NOT one of the methods of recording data in a patient's medical record?
a. Physician enters data.
b. Medical assistant dictates data.
c. Physician dictates data.
d. Physician keys data.

53. The patient's case history will include all of the following elements, except
a. past family history.
b. chief complaint.
c. history of present illness.
d. insurance history.

_____ 54. The review of systems is a/an
   a. inventory of body systems obtained through a series of questions.
   b. physical examination.
   c. examination of all body systems.
   d. review of the family history of all family members.

_____ 55. The probable outcome of the disease or injury and the prospect of recovery is called the
   a. diagnosis.   c. treatment.
   b. prognosis.   d. progress.

_____ 56. A medical assistant may need to abstract data from the patient's medical record in order to complete a/an
   a. ledger.   c. insurance form.
   b. external audit.   d. review of systems.

_____ 57. If unusual billing patterns occur, the government or insurance carrier may perform a/an
   a. internal review.   c. abstraction.
   b. authentication visit.   d. external audit.

_____ 58. The diagnosis is also called the
   a. impression.   c. treatment.
   b. management.   d. prognosis.

_____ 59. Which record system files all documents in chronologic order without regard to their source?
   a. Problem-oriented   c. Integrated
   b. Source-oriented   d. Medical

_____ 60. Type, depth, site, and percentage of total body surface are important in documenting
   a. burns.   c. lacerations.
   b. lesions.   d. fractures.

_____ 61. The proprietary or trade name of a drug as copyrighted by the manufacturer is known as the
   a. generic name.   c. brand name.
   b. chemical name.   d. pharmacy name.

_____ 62. Rubbing an ointment into the skin for absorption is an example of
   a. inhalation.   c. inunction.
   b. injection.   d. instillation.

_____ 63. Intra-articular, intradermal, intramuscular, and subcutaneous are all examples of
   a. inhalations.   c. inunctions.
   b. injection routes.   d. instillations.

_____ 64. Vaporizers and nebulizers are examples of apparatus used to administer medication by means of
   a. inhalation.   c. inunction.
   b. injection.   d. instillation.

_____ 65. Ointments, creams, and liniments are all examples of
   a. transdermal medications.   c. oral substances.
   b. parenteral medications.   d. topical substances.

_____ 66. All methods of giving medications by means of a needle or cannula through the skin are referred to as
   a. transdermal.   c. topical.
   b. parenteral.   d. sublingual.

_____ 67. A nicotine patch is an example of

a. transdermal delivery.
c. topical delivery.
b. parenteral delivery.
d. sublingual delivery.

68. If a patient taking medication calls with symptoms of dizziness, drowsiness, nausea, and vomiting, the medical assistant should immediately
    a. tell the patient to stop the medication.
    b. bring the situation to the physician's attention.
    c. disregard these symptoms as cause for alarm.
    d. tell the patient to wait 2 hours and call back with an update.

69. A vitamin is an example of a
    a. placebo.
    c. stimulant.
    b. sedative.
    d. prophylactic.

70. What may be given as a control in pharmaceutical studies of drugs?
    a. Placebo
    c. Stimulant
    b. Sedative
    d. Prophylactic

71. What is the correct term for a preparation with undissolved ingredients that must be shaken well before using?
    a. Solution
    c. Stimulant
    b. Suspension
    d. Antiseptic

72. What is the correct term for a liquid with ingredients dissolved evenly?
    a. Antiseptic
    c. Stimulant
    b. Suspension
    d. Solution

73. A vasoconstrictor causes
    a. increased secretion.
    c. dilation of blood vessels.
    b. constriction of blood vessels.
    d. decreased secretion.

74. What is the name of the federal law passed in 1970 that requires the pharmaceutical industry to maintain physical security and strict record keeping for intoxicating drugs?
    a. The Volstead Act
    c. The Controlled Substances Act
    b. The Food, Drug, and Cosmetic Act
    d. The Marijuana Tax Act

75. What is another name for the National Prohibition Act, which prohibited manufacture, transportation, and sale of beverages containing more than 0.5% alcohol?
    a. The Food, Drug, and Cosmetic Act
    c. The Volstead Act
    b. The Harrison Act
    d. The Marijuana Tax Act

76. Which drugs in the Schedule of Controlled Substances have the highest potential for abuse?
    a. Schedule V drugs
    c. Schedule II drugs
    b. Schedule IV drugs
    d. Schedule I drugs

77. The standard "signature component" of a prescription refers to
    a. the physician's signature.
    c. instructions to the patient.
    b. instructions to the pharmacist.
    d. the patient's signature.

78. The standard "subscription component" of a prescription refers to the
    a. instructions to the patient.
    c. name and strength of the medication.
    b. directions to the pharmacist.
    d. word recipe.

79. The standard "inscription component" of a prescription refers to the
    a. name, quantity, and strength of the drug.
    b. physician's signature.

c. instructions to the patient.

d. directions to the pharmacist.

_____ 80. When a patient calls the office requesting a medication refill, the medical assistant should find out:
a. the name of the medication.
b. the dosage and strength.
c. the number of tablets/capsules.
d. all of the above.

_____ 81. Interoffice memorandums generally
a. are informal in tone.
b. are formal in tone.
c. include confidential matters.
d. are not proofread as carefully.

_____ 82. Which type of office memorandum gives brief instructions?
a. Informative
b. Directive
c. Administrative
d. Form

_____ 83. Which type of memorandum states policy or judgment on a specific topic?
a. Informative
b. Directive
c. Administrative
d. Form

_____ 84. Use a spell checker for _____.
a. all proofreading
b. correcting word usage and grammar
c. obvious errors only
d. never use a spell checker

_____ 85. A letter should not be mailed if it
a. has unbalanced margins.
b. has a misspelled word.
c. has an abbreviated city name.
d. contains any of the above

_____ 86. What part of the letter contains the message to be conveyed to the recipient?
a. Subject line
b. Postscript
c. Body
d. Salutation

_____ 87. What type of notation is used to indicate that separate material is attached?
a. Copy
b. Enclosure
c. Reference
d. Attention

_____ 88. "Dear Dr. Jones" is an example of a/an
a. complimentary close.
b. signature line.
c. salutation.
d. attention line.

_____ 89. "Sincerely" is an example of a
a. complimentary close.
b. salutation.
c. signature line.
d. title line.

_____ 90. "Director, Medical Research" is an example of a
a. signature line.
b. title line.
c. salutation.
d. reference.

_____ 91. "cc: Dr. Robert Smith" is an example of a/an
a. enclosure notation.
b. signature line.
c. attention line.
d. copy notation.

_____ 92. Which term describes a word processing software option that allows you to see how the document will look when it is printed?
a. Print preview
b. Cut and paste
c. Grammar check
d. Letterhead

_____ 93. What may be used as a guide to create a document, which often has basic headings, saves keystrokes, and speeds generating a document or report?

a. Thesaurus
b. Form letter
c. Template
d. Copyedit

94. Two styles of letter punctuation are
    a. modified and simplified.
    b. open and mixed.
    c. closed and open.
    d. mixed and modified.

95. What is the time frame in which correspondence should be answered?
    a. Within 24 hours
    b. Within two days
    c. Within five days
    d. Within one week

96. What is the correct term for an afterthought which is keyed after the last line of a letter?
    a. Notation
    b. Attention line
    c. Postscript
    d. Enclosure line

97. A well-written letter will conclude
    a. on a positive note.
    b. with jargon.
    c. with a joke.
    d. with reference to another document.

98. An electronic typewriter typically has
    a. many font types and sizes available.
    b. only one type size.
    c. several sizes but no different fonts.
    d. two type sizes.

99. Standard or expedited services such as global airmail and global express mail are examples of delivery options offered by the USPS for
    a. express mail.
    b. international mail.
    c. priority mail.
    d. registered mail.

100. The fastest and most reliable delivery service offered by the USPS is
    a. media mail.
    b. express mail.
    c. certified mail.
    d. parcel post.

101. It is best to send mail with a declared value, such as checks, money, or valuable merchandise, by
    a. special mail.
    b. registered mail.
    c. certified mail.
    d. first class mail.

102. In a medical office, when it is necessary to prove that a piece of mail has been delivered, such as for collection purposes, letters of dismissal of a patient, or other situations, what type of service is used?
    a. Special delivery
    b. Registered mail
    c. Certified mail
    d. Priority mail

103. Which of the following statements regarding business e-mail etiquette is accurate?
    a. It is acceptable to express humor and anger in e-mail.
    b. E-mail is considered the employee's property when he uses it.
    c. Company e-mail is company property.
    d. It is best if you use all capital letters to make an e-mail easier to read.

104. When operating a fax machine,
    a. it is all right to leave staples and paper clips in the document as it runs through the machine.
    b. pull the paper out by hand to interrupt transmittal of a document.
    c. try to transmit at times of the day when telephone rates are least expensive.
    d. the fax can be sent to any phone number.

105. When handling faxed records,
    a. keep a fax report of all transmissions indicating the date, time, and destination.

b. it is safe to fax financial information.

c. psychiatric records should be faxed to expedite treatment.

d. do not adhere to confidentiality rules because fax machines are always kept in confidential locations.

_____106. When addressing an envelope for optical character recognition,
a. all characters should be typed in lower case letters and double spaced.
b. the ZIP code should precede the two-letter state abbreviation.
c. eliminate punctuation marks.
d. type the address as close to the bottom of the envelope as possible.

_____107. The USPS has many services available online, including
a. ZIP code look up.   c. stamp purchasing.
b. postage calculation.   d. all of the above.

_____108. In a ZIP + 4 code, the last four digits speed mail delivery by specifying
a. one of the 10 areas of the United States.   c. a sectional center.
b. a city block, building, or P.O. box.   d. a post office.

_____109. Suspicious characteristics of mail include
a. signs of leakage.   c. ticking sounds.
b. protruding wires.   d. all of the above.

_____110. A mail classification that includes thick envelopes, tubes, and packages is
a. registered mail.   c. periodicals.
b. media mail.   d. parcel post.

_____111. The name of the form used which indicates the name and address of the sender and addressee and shows proof that a special communication was sent by a deadline is
a. registered letter receipt.   c. certificate of mailing.
b. express mail acknowledgement.   d. tracking form.

_____112. When sending mail to a foreign country, on the last line of the envelope type the address in capital letters of the
a. recipient's name.   c. country's full name.
b. country abbreviation.   d. country code.

_____113. When mail has two delivery addresses indicated, the mail is delivered to the address that
a. appears directly above the city, state, and zip code line.
b. is closest to the top of the envelope.
c. appears as a street address.
d. appears as a post office box.

_____114. What special notation is used when the sender would like mail to be sent on to the addressee's new address?
a. Address service requested   c. Change service requested
b. Return service requested   d. Forward service requested

_____115. What should each letter be checked for before sealing the envelope?
a. Written signature   c. Both a and b
b. Any necessary enclosures   d. Neither a nor b

_____116. E-mail can create self-documenting medical records, improve time management, and enrich the provider-patient relationship for
a. the patient.   c. the medical assistant.

b. the physician.

d. none of the above.

_____117. When unsolicited or unknown e-mail is received, care should be taken before opening it because you could expose the computer system to
a. persons of unknown origin.
b. viruses.

c. subscriptions.
d. unauthorized access.

_____118. Assume that all e-mail messages are
a. kept forever.
b. deleted before being read.

c. not legal.
d. your property.

_____119. E-mail signature lines should contain
a. an inspirational quote.
b. as much information as you would like.

c. the employee's name only.
d. no more than six lines.

_____120. Fax communication can be used
a. to refill prescriptions.
b. to resubmit unpaid insurance claims.

c. to obtain preauthorizations.
d. for any of the above.

Matching

Match each term with the correct statement below.
a. abstract
b. attending physician
c. audit
d. case history
e. consulting physician

f. diagnosis
g. flow sheet
h. laboratory report
i. medical record
j. medical report

_____121. extracting information from parts of the medical record to complete a form
_____122. record kept that tracks a specific disease, condition, or test result over time
_____123. a clinical record showing the names of tests performed in a laboratory and test results
_____124. the determination of a disease or injury
_____125. to conduct a review of records
_____126. provider whose opinion or advice is requested
_____127. provider who is legally responsible for the care and treatment given to a patient
_____128. permanent legal document formally stating the results of an examination

Match each term with the correct statement below.
a. objective
b. ordering physician
c. prognosis
d. progress report
e. referring physician

f. sign
g. subjective
h. symptom
i. treating physician
j. x-ray report

_____129. information apparent to the observer
_____130. objective evidence typically associated with a given condition
_____131. written radiographic findings
_____132. any morbid phenomenon, condition, or evidence of disease

_____133. forecast of the outcome of a disease or injury

_____134. any information that the patient provides to the physician, describing subjective information such as pain

_____135. written observations made at examinations of a patient subsequent to an initial examination

_____136. provider who sends the patient for testing or treatment

_____137. provider directing the selection, preparation, or administration of tests, medication, or treatment

Match each term with the correct statement below.

a. analgesic
b. antacid
c. bronchodilator
d. decongestant
e. diuretic
f. emetic
g. hemostatic
h. laxative
i. miotic

j. narcotic
k. ointment
l. tranquilizer
m. brand name
n. chemical name
o. Drug Enforcement Administration
p. generic name
q. prescription
r. Food and Drug Administration

_____138. drug used to control bleeding

_____139. drug that reduces anxiety without clouding consciousness; a sedative

_____140. drug that increases the excretion of urine

_____141. drug that causes vomiting

_____142. soft, fatty substance having soothing or healing action

_____143. drug that relieves pain and produces sleep or stupor

_____144. drug used to dilate bronchial tubes

_____145. drug that decreases congestion or swelling

_____146. drug that neutralizes acidity, especially in the digestive tract

_____147. agency that regulates the manufacturing and dispensing of dangerous drugs

_____148. indicates the chemical content of the drug

_____149. indicates ownership by a manufacturer and serves as a trademark

_____150. gives premarket approval for all new drugs

_____151. established, nonproprietary name

_____152. order to prepare medications

Match each term with the correct statement below.

a. edit
b. elite type
c. ergonomics
d. form letter
e. full block letter style
f. interoffice memorandum
g. mixed punctuation
h. modified block letter style
i. open punctuation

j. photocopy
k. photocopy machine
l. pica type
m. proofreading
n. simplified letter style
o. thesaurus
p. transcriptionist
q. word processing
r. word processing log

_____153. type size measuring 12 characters to the horizontal inch

_____154. letter formatted with all lines flush with the left margin
_____155. standardized letter; also called "repetitive letter"
_____156. written message circulated within an organization
_____157. record of all word processing work used to find documents quickly and easily
_____158. letter formatted with the date and closing lines beginning at the center
_____159. term designating the reproduction of original documents
_____160. duplicating machine that copies material onto paper in a few seconds
_____161. system using computerized and text-editing equipment to produce printed letters, reports, and other office documents
_____162. person who converts recorded dictation to hard copy
_____163. punctuation style using colon or comma after salutation and complimentary close
_____164. science of designing office systems to meet the needs of the human body
_____165. carefully scanning the final document to catch errors and make corrections
_____166. any type of correction, alteration, or refinement of a document
_____167. punctuation style using no punctuation mark used after salutation or complimentary close
_____168. letter style which eliminates both the salutation and the complimentary close

Match each term with the correct statement below.

a. annotate
b. bar code sorter (BCS)
c. certified mail
d. domestic mail
e. electronic mail
f. enclosure
g. facsimile (fax) communication
h. mail classification
i. mail log
j. registered mail
k. service endorsement
l. zone improvement plan (ZIP + 4)

_____169. notification to the postal service on the envelope stating what is to be done with undelivered mail
_____170. nine-digit code on the envelope
_____171. a mail service determination based on contents, weight, destination, and speed of delivery
_____172. electronic process for transmitting written communications via telecommunication lines
_____173. computerized process of sending, receiving, storing, and forwarding messages and memos digitally
_____174. supplemental item contained in an envelope with written communication
_____175. mail delivered in the United States, Canada, and Mexico
_____176. first-class mail service that provides, for a fee, a record that mail has been delivered and guarantees an indemnity if it is not received
_____177. detailed record of incoming and outgoing mail activity
_____178. to make explanatory notations in the margins on medical correspondence so that actions can be taken
_____179. code imprinted on first-class mail to speed sorting and delivery
_____180. postal service that provides, for a fee, a receipt to the sender of first-class mail and a record of its delivery

Completion
Complete each statement.

181. In the context of medical records handling, to _____ means to extract or pull out information from a patient's chart.

182. The acronym SOAP stands for _____ complaints, _____ findings, _____ of status, and diagnostic or therapeutic _____.

183. SOAP and CHEDDAR are methods of structuring _____ _____.

184. An advantage of the _____ record system is that it allows the physician to find and compare information quickly.

185. Entries in the patient's record must be as _____ as possible.

186. The _____ record system is the most common paper-based system, but it does not provide a quick overall picture of the patient's health.

187. All individuals who provide health care services may be known as _____ because they record facts and observations about the patient and the patient's health.

188. A physician's _____ after the typed note indicates that the entry is true and correct at the time of writing and makes the chart admissible as evidence in court.

189. The physician may use a/an _____ of the body area in order to document a problem and where it has occurred. This should also be kept in the chart, dated, and signed.

190. In medical records, it is acceptable to use standard _____ and _____ that are commonly understood and can be decoded by the general medical community.

191. HEENT stands for _____, _____, _____, _____, and _____.

192. If incorrect data occurs in a computerized medical record, never _____ or _____ _____ the error.

193. The _____ history is an age-appropriate review of activities and occupation.

194. The levels of Evaluation and Management (E/M) services are based on four types of history: _____ focused, _____ _____ focused, _____, and _____.

195. The federal agency that issues narcotic and hypnotic licenses to physicians is called the _____ _____ _____.

196. _____ - _____ - _____ drugs, also referred to as nonprescription drugs, may be evaluated by the FDA and released to be purchased without a prescription.

197. A person skilled in the art or practice of preparing, preserving, compounding, and dispensing drugs is a/an _____.

198. A large comprehensive reference book used by physicians and medical assistants to find information about prescription drugs is the _____ _____ _____.

199. The expiration date of medications should be checked periodically in order to ensure that they have not exceeded their _____ _____.

200. _____ _____ are solid, liquid, or gas wastes that can cause death, illness, or injury to people or destruction of the environment if improperly discarded.

201. In the physician's office, a prime target of drug abusers is the _____ _____, which must not be left lying around.

202. The assistant must be aware that medication taken in the correct dosage can still produce _____ _____.

203. A/an _____ reaction can be caused when some medications are taken in conjunction with others.

204. Every time medication is prescribed, a patient should be asked if they have any medication _____.

205. A/an _____ _____ should be placed on the patient's medical record if they have ever had an adverse side effect to any medication.

206. _____ are a suspension of infectious agents used to convey resistance to infectious diseases.

207. A/an _____ _____ can be given to patients to help keep track of the name and dosage of drugs, as well as time(s) of day they should be taken.

208. A/an _____ _____, also called a drug flow sheet, is kept in the medical office to track frequency of drug refills.

209. A/An _____ _____ letter style, formatted with date, closing, and writer's information aligned at the center has a more balanced appearance.

210. The two most traditional type styles for electronic typewriters are _____ and _____.

211. A letter should not be mailed if it has a word incorrectly _____ at the end of the typing line.

212. All correspondence should be accurate, _____, _____, and _____.

213. _____ _____ on a computer move the cursor up, down, left, and right.

214. _____ _____ perform delete and search operations.

215. A well-written letter should appeal to the _____ point of view.

216. Use _____ language when writing a letter to a familiar person.

217. A letter will create a favorable impression if it arouses the reader's interest with the first _____.

218. A/an _____ is an alphabetic listing of synonyms and antonyms used to find alternative words.

219. The _____ of a letter should deal immediately with the subject matter in a friendly and courteous manner.

220. In order to avoid offending the recipient, be careful to use _____-neutral terms.

221. An ergonomic workstation is adjustable for proper computer-operator position to avoid _____ or strain to the body.

222. The USPS device that can read and process mail at the speed of 36,000 pieces per hour is known as _____ _____ _____.

223. A/An _____ _____ is used to determine the weight of mail.

224. The USPS toll-free line or online services can help calculate _____ _____ for commonly used mail services if the weight of the item is known.

225. To check accuracy of a postal scale, weigh _____ _____ on it. They should weigh one ounce.

226. A/An _____ _____ is used to print prepaid postage directly onto envelopes or packages.

227. When handling a large volume of mail, it is advisable to put on _____ _____ if you have open cuts or skin lesions on your hands.

228. If suspicious mail is opened, you should notify your _____ and local _____ _____ _____ immediately.

229. When opening mail, a single small _____ may be stapled to the front of a letter, but a large attachment is usually fastened to the back.

230. After opening _____, the medical assistant should check the contents to determine that nothing is missing or broken.

231. It is vital to know how to handle _____ mail safely since the increase of terrorist activity in the United States.

232. The USPS offers _____ _____ to track mail, provide proof of mailing, and ensure delivery. The level of tracking will determine which service to use.

233. _____ delivery assures that only a specified person will receive a piece of mail.

234. The bottom right-hand corner of an envelope is the space reserved for the _____ _____ that is printed during OCR processing.

235. Although the USPS accepts any color combination of ink and paper, _____ ink on _____ paper is most easily read and processed by OCR.

236. When both a street address and a post office box number are included in an address, it is best to use the _____ _____ _____ _____.

237. _____ _____ are used to request a new address and to provide the USPS with instructions on how to handle undeliverable mail.

238. _____ envelopes are popular because they eliminate the need to type an address twice.

239. It is essential to remember that the patient must sign a/an _____ _____ in order for communication to take place via e-mail.

240. Court cases regarding issues of privacy and ownership in electronic communication systems indicate that e-mail is _____ property.

Short Answer

241. Describe the proper method for correcting a typed or handwritten medical record entry.

242. List the four levels of complexity in medical decision making.

243. Describe the difference between subjective and objective information.

244. What is the difference between a Schedule I drug and a Schedule V drug?

245. Why are some prescription abbreviations prohibited by JCAHO?

246. Demonstrate the vertical and horizontal formats for the main headings of memorandums.

247. Describe what each of the main headings in a memorandum should contain.

248. List four references that are useful to have for letter writing.

249. Name three characteristics of a well-written letter.

250. Name two delivery services that compete with the U.S. Postal Service.

Exam 3
Answer Section

TRUE/FALSE

1.	ANS: T	PTS: 1
2.	ANS: T	PTS: 1
3.	ANS: T	PTS: 1
4.	ANS: F	PTS: 1
5.	ANS: F	PTS: 1
6.	ANS: T	PTS: 1
7.	ANS: T	PTS: 1
8.	ANS: T	PTS: 1
9.	ANS: F	PTS: 1
10.	ANS: F	PTS: 1
11.	ANS: F	PTS: 1
12.	ANS: T	PTS: 1
13.	ANS: T	PTS: 1
14.	ANS: F	PTS: 1
15.	ANS: F	PTS: 1
16.	ANS: T	PTS: 1
17.	ANS: F	PTS: 1
18.	ANS: T	PTS: 1
19.	ANS: F	PTS: 1
20.	ANS: T	PTS: 1
21.	ANS: F	PTS: 1
22.	ANS: F	PTS: 1
23.	ANS: T	PTS: 1
24.	ANS: F	PTS: 1
25.	ANS: T	PTS: 1
26.	ANS: F	PTS: 1
27.	ANS: F	PTS: 1
28.	ANS: F	PTS: 1
29.	ANS: T	PTS: 1
30.	ANS: F	PTS: 1
31.	ANS: F	PTS: 1
32.	ANS: T	PTS: 1
33.	ANS: T	PTS: 1
34.	ANS: T	PTS: 1
35.	ANS: F	PTS: 1
36.	ANS: F	PTS: 1
37.	ANS: T	PTS: 1

38.	ANS: F	PTS: 1
39.	ANS: T	PTS: 1
40.	ANS: F	PTS: 1

MULTIPLE CHOICE

41.	ANS: D	PTS: 1
42.	ANS: C	PTS: 1
43.	ANS: B	PTS: 1
44.	ANS: A	PTS: 1
45.	ANS: D	PTS: 1
46.	ANS: C	PTS: 1
47.	ANS: A	PTS: 1
48.	ANS: B	PTS: 1
49.	ANS: A	PTS: 1
50.	ANS: D	PTS: 1
51.	ANS: C	PTS: 1
52.	ANS: B	PTS: 1
53.	ANS: D	PTS: 1
54.	ANS: A	PTS: 1
55.	ANS: B	PTS: 1
56.	ANS: C	PTS: 1
57.	ANS: D	PTS: 1
58.	ANS: A	PTS: 1
59.	ANS: C	PTS: 1
60.	ANS: A	PTS: 1
61.	ANS: C	PTS: 1
62.	ANS: C	PTS: 1
63.	ANS: B	PTS: 1
64.	ANS: A	PTS: 1
65.	ANS: D	PTS: 1
66.	ANS: B	PTS: 1
67.	ANS: A	PTS: 1
68.	ANS: B	PTS: 1
69.	ANS: D	PTS: 1
70.	ANS: A	PTS: 1
71.	ANS: B	PTS: 1
72.	ANS: D	PTS: 1
73.	ANS: B	PTS: 1
74.	ANS: C	PTS: 1
75.	ANS: A	PTS: 1
76.	ANS: D	PTS: 1
77.	ANS: C	PTS: 1

78.	ANS: B	PTS: 1
79.	ANS: A	PTS: 1
80.	ANS: D	PTS: 1
81.	ANS: A	PTS: 1
82.	ANS: B	PTS: 1
83.	ANS: C	PTS: 1
84.	ANS: C	PTS: 1
85.	ANS: D	PTS: 1
86.	ANS: C	PTS: 1
87.	ANS: B	PTS: 1
88.	ANS: C	PTS: 1
89.	ANS: A	PTS: 1
90.	ANS: B	PTS: 1
91.	ANS: D	PTS: 1
92.	ANS: A	PTS: 1
93.	ANS: C	PTS: 1
94.	ANS: B	PTS: 1
95.	ANS: A	PTS: 1
96.	ANS: C	PTS: 1
97.	ANS: A	PTS: 1
98.	ANS: D	PTS: 1
99.	ANS: B	PTS: 1
100.	ANS: B	PTS: 1
101.	ANS: B	PTS: 1
102.	ANS: C	PTS: 1
103.	ANS: C	PTS: 1
104.	ANS: C	PTS: 1
105.	ANS: A	PTS: 1
106.	ANS: C	PTS: 1
107.	ANS: D	PTS: 1
108.	ANS: B	PTS: 1
109.	ANS: D	PTS: 1
110.	ANS: D	PTS: 1
111.	ANS: C	PTS: 1
112.	ANS: C	PTS: 1
113.	ANS: A	PTS: 1
114.	ANS: D	PTS: 1
115.	ANS: C	PTS: 1
116.	ANS: B	PTS: 1
117.	ANS: B	PTS: 1
118.	ANS: A	PTS: 1
119.	ANS: D	PTS: 1
120.	ANS: D	PTS: 1

MATCHING

121. ANS: A   PTS: 1
122. ANS: G   PTS: 1
123. ANS: H   PTS: 1
124. ANS: F   PTS: 1
125. ANS: C   PTS: 1
126. ANS: E   PTS: 1
127. ANS: B   PTS: 1
128. ANS: J   PTS: 1

129. ANS: A   PTS: 1
130. ANS: F   PTS: 1
131. ANS: J   PTS: 1
132. ANS: H   PTS: 1
133. ANS: C   PTS: 1
134. ANS: G   PTS: 1
135. ANS: D   PTS: 1
136. ANS: E   PTS: 1
137. ANS: B   PTS: 1

138. ANS: G   PTS: 1
139. ANS: L   PTS: 1
140. ANS: E   PTS: 1
141. ANS: F   PTS: 1
142. ANS: K   PTS: 1
143. ANS: J   PTS: 1
144. ANS: C   PTS: 1
145. ANS: D   PTS: 1
146. ANS: B   PTS: 1
147. ANS: O   PTS: 1
148. ANS: N   PTS: 1
149. ANS: M   PTS: 1
150. ANS: R   PTS: 1
151. ANS: P   PTS: 1
152. ANS: Q   PTS: 1

153. ANS: B   PTS: 1
154. ANS: E   PTS: 1
155. ANS: D   PTS: 1
156. ANS: F   PTS: 1
157. ANS: R   PTS: 1

158. ANS: H   PTS: 1
159. ANS: J   PTS: 1
160. ANS: K   PTS: 1
161. ANS: Q   PTS: 1
162. ANS: P   PTS: 1
163. ANS: G   PTS: 1
164. ANS: C   PTS: 1
165. ANS: M   PTS: 1
166. ANS: A   PTS: 1
167. ANS: I   PTS: 1
168. ANS: N   PTS: 1

169. ANS: K   PTS: 1
170. ANS: L   PTS: 1
171. ANS: H   PTS: 1
172. ANS: G   PTS: 1
173. ANS: E   PTS: 1
174. ANS: F   PTS: 1
175. ANS: D   PTS: 1
176. ANS: J   PTS: 1
177. ANS: I   PTS: 1
178. ANS: A   PTS: 1
179. ANS: B   PTS: 1
180. ANS: C   PTS: 1

COMPLETION

181. ANS: abstract

    PTS: 1
182. ANS: subjective, objective, assessment, plan

    PTS: 1
183. ANS:
    progress notes
    chart notes

    PTS: 1
184. ANS: problem-oriented

    PTS: 1
185. ANS: legible

    PTS: 1

186. ANS: source-oriented

     PTS: 1
187. ANS: documenters

     PTS: 1
188. ANS: signature

     PTS: 1
189. ANS: illustration

     PTS: 1
190. ANS: acronyms, abbreviations

     PTS: 1
191. ANS: head, eyes, ears, nose, throat

     PTS: 1
192. ANS: delete, key over

     PTS: 1
193. ANS: social

     PTS: 1
194. ANS: problem, expanded problem, detailed, comprehensive

     PTS: 1
195. ANS:
     Drug Enforcement Agency
     DEA

     PTS: 1
196. ANS:
     Over-the-counter
     OTC

     PTS: 1
197. ANS: pharmacist

     PTS: 1
198. ANS:
     Physicians' Desk Reference
     PDR

     PTS: 1

199. ANS: shelf life

PTS: 1
200. ANS: Hazardous wastes

PTS: 1
201. ANS: prescription pad

PTS: 1
202. ANS: side effects

PTS: 1
203. ANS: adverse

PTS: 1
204. ANS: allergies

PTS: 1
205. ANS: alert tag

PTS: 1
206. ANS: Vaccines

PTS: 1
207. ANS: medication schedule

PTS: 1
208. ANS: medication log

PTS: 1
209. ANS: modified block

PTS: 1
210. ANS: pica, elite

PTS: 1
211. ANS: divided

PTS: 1
212. ANS: clear, concise, complete

PTS: 1
213. ANS: Directional keys

PTS: 1

214. ANS: Function keys

   PTS: 1
215. ANS: reader's

   PTS: 1
216. ANS:
   conversational
   informal

   PTS: 1
217. ANS: sentence

   PTS: 1
218. ANS: thesaurus

   PTS: 1
219. ANS:
   introduction
   first paragraph

   PTS: 1
220. ANS: gender

   PTS: 1
221. ANS: injury

   PTS: 1
222. ANS:
   optical character recognition
   OCR

   PTS: 1
223. ANS: postal scale

   PTS: 1
224. ANS: postage costs

   PTS: 1
225. ANS:
   nine pennies
   9 pennies

   PTS: 1
226. ANS: postage meter

PTS: 1

227. ANS: disposable gloves

PTS: 1

228. ANS: supervisor, law enforcement authorities

PTS: 1

229. ANS: enclosure

PTS: 1

230. ANS: packages

PTS: 1

231. ANS: suspicious

PTS: 1

232. ANS: special services

PTS: 1

233. ANS: Restricted

PTS: 1

234. ANS: bar code

PTS: 1

235. ANS: black, white

PTS: 1

236. ANS: post office box number

PTS: 1

237. ANS: Service endorsements

PTS: 1

238. ANS: Window

PTS: 1

239. ANS: consent form

PTS: 1

240. ANS: company

PTS: 1

SHORT ANSWER

241. ANS:
Draw a line through the incorrect entry so it remains readable. Insert the correct information above, below, or in the margin near the original entry. The person making the correction writes "corr.," the date, and their initials in the margin.

PTS: 1

242. ANS:
Straightforward (SF)
Low Complexity (LC)
Moderate Complexity (MC)
High Complexity (HC)

PTS: 1

243. ANS:
Subjective information comes from the patient's statements about their feelings or symptoms experienced. Objective information comes from anything the physician has seen, heard, felt, or measured.

PTS: 1

244. ANS:
Schedule I drugs are most easily abused and habit forming. Schedule V drugs are less dangerous to the user and are not subject to as much abuse

PTS: 1

245. ANS:
For the safety of the patient; some abbreviations are easily misunderstood, misread, or misinterpreted.

PTS: 1

246. ANS:
Vertical   DATE:
               TO:
               FROM:
               SUBJECT:

Horizontal   TO: DATE:
               FROM: SUBJECT:

PTS: 1

247. ANS:
DATE: Date the message originated. TO: Alphabetic list of all names of persons or departments for routing; titles not necessary. FROM: Name of the writer or dictator. SUBJECT: Summary of main points.

PTS: 1

248. ANS:
English grammar reference book
medical dictionary
thesaurus
secretarial manual of style and format

PTS: 1

249. ANS:
Any of the following three answers:
a. creates a favorable impression by arousing the reader's interest with the first sentence
b. appeals to the reader's point of view
c. correct in every grammatical detail
d. courteous, friendly, and sincere, promoting goodwill
e. accurate, clear, concise, and complete
f. flows smoothly and concludes by telling the reader how to respond
g. avoids jargon and stilted phrases
h. concludes on a positive note

PTS: 1

250. ANS:

Any two of the following (others may be indicated):
United Parcel Service
Federal Express
DHL WorldWide Express

PTS: 1

Exam 4

True/False
Indicate whether the statement is true or false.

_____ 1. Federal regulations prohibit a physician from establishing more than one fee schedule.

_____ 2. The Fair Debt Collections Practices Act states that telephone calls for collection activities should be placed after 8:00 a.m. and before 9:00 p.m.

_____ 3. Financial transactions are those that involve only cash.

_____ 4. If the endorser's name is incorrect on the face of the check, it should be endorsed twice.

_____ 5. A paycheck presented in payment of the patient's medical bill is an example of a third-party check.

_____ 6. Federal law prohibits a retailer from converting a paper check into an electronic check.

_____ 7. Point-of-sale banking is a system that brings banking to the business location, allowing instant transfer of funds.

_____ 8. Most medical practices rely on the administrative medical assistant to manage bookkeeping transactions accurately.

_____ 9. An industrial accident or disease is a foreseeable event arising out of one's employment.

_____ 10. The patient's insurance identification card indicates the patient's premium.

_____ 11. A referral is the same as a consultation.

_____ 12. The job of office manager may include delegating certain duties.

_____ 13. Encouraging specialization within the medical office will decrease office productivity.

_____ 14. Cross-training staff decreases efficiency.

_____ 15. A system of controlling inventory is important in order to maintain an adequate number of office supplies.

_____ 16. A profit or loss statement is a financial report for a specific employee indicating how much money that employee generated for the medical office.

_____ 17. A federal minimum wage amount is set for all employees 21 years in age or older.

_____ 18. Do not answer questions about your personal life unless the answer will demonstrate an ability to perform the job.

_____ 19. The interviewer should not ask questions about the interviewee's provisions for child care.

_____ 20. It is not necessary for an employer to keep verification that you are eligible for employment in the United States.

Multiple Choice
Identify the choice that best completes the statement or answers the question.

_____ 21. What is the method called which divides patient accounts by alphabet, account number, insurance type, or calendar day of first visit in order to send monthly statements in a more even distribution?
a. Cycle billing
b. Open accounts
c. Aging accounts
d. Monthly billing

_____ 22. The state of being legally unable to pay one's debts is known as
a. credit.
b. delinquency.
c. bankruptcy.
d. billing.

_____ 23. "Trust" in regard to financial obligations is known as
a. bankruptcy.
b. credit.
c. faith.
d. petition.

_____ 24. Fees for professional services rendered are called
a. quantum merit.
b. debits.
c. charges.
d. credits.

_____ 25. A common-law principle that means the patient promises to pay the physician as much as she deserves for labor is known as

a. quantum merit.   c. fee-for-service.
b. credit law.   d. local labor laws.

26. What is the name of the act that states if a physician agrees to extend credit to one patient, the same financial arrangement must be extended to all patients who request it?
a. The Fair Debt Collection Practices Act
b. The Equal Credit Opportunity Act
c. The Federal Truth in Lending Act
d. The Fair Credit Billing Act

27. Which act governs anyone who charges interest or agrees to more than four payments for a given service?
a. The Fair Debt Collection Practices Act
b. The Equal Credit Opportunity Act
c. The Federal Truth in Lending Act
d. The Fair Credit Billing Act

28. What is the name for records of business transactions on the books that represent unsecured accounts receivable where credit has been extended without a formal written contract?
a. Physician accounts   c. Closed accounts
b. Open-book accounts   d. Written-contract accounts

29. An analysis of accounts receivable indicating 60, 90, and 120 days past due is called
a. accounts receivable control.   c. aging accounts.
b. open-ended accounts.   d. monthly statements.

30. What may a physician offer patients paying cash, as long as she offers it to all patients?
a. Credit   c. Insurance discounts
b. Debit   d. Discounts

31. Which fee schedule involves three columns, a participating fee, a nonparticipating fee, and a limiting charge?
a. Professional fee schedule   c. Managed care fee schedule
b. Medicare fee schedule   d. Private insurance fee schedule

32. What is the name of the document that is a combination form that can be used as a bill, an insurance form, and a routing document?
a. Patient instructional sheet   c. Multipurpose billing form
b. Form letter   d. Itemized statement

33. What is the name for a phrase which appears on the billing statement to promote payment?
a. Dun message   c. Credit message
b. Aging message   d. Billing message

34. What service may be employed by a medical practice to prepare and send all monthly statements and to place collection calls if necessary?
a. Collection agency   c. Credit counselor
b. Billing service   d. Clearinghouse

35. When a patient pays for medical services directly, then requests reimbursement from the insurance company to be sent to themselves, it is called a/an
a. billing service.   c. third-party reimbursement.
b. credit counseling service.   d. individual responsibility program.

36. According to the Fair Debt Collection Practices Act,
a. debtors may be contacted only once a day.

b. debtors may not be contacted on Sunday or the Sabbath.

c. postcards are not allowed for collection purposes.

d. all of the above.

_____ 37. Complete the statement, "The longer an account remains delinquent,
a. the easier it will be to collect."
b. the harder it will be to collect."
c. the more effective a collection agency will be."
d. the more money the physician will make."

_____ 38. If the patient sends an unsigned check for payment on an account, you should
a. ask them to come in to the office to sign the check.
b. send them an envelope so they can send a new check.
c. verify their name and address and send a new bill.
d. ask for immediate payment.

_____ 39. If unable to trace and contact a patient, turn the account over to a collection agency
a. within 30 days. c. immediately.
b. in a week. d. at the next billing cycle.

_____ 40. A check must be written as payable to the
a. payee. c. bearer.
b. drawer. d. maker.

_____ 41. The person who signs a check or order to the bank to pay funds from an account is the
a. bearer. c. payee.
b. drawer. d. drawee.

_____ 42. What is the name of the document that is purchased for face value plus a fee and is issued according to the purchaser's instructions and signed by the purchaser?
a. Money order c. Automatic transfer
b. Bank draft d. Certified check

_____ 43. Removal of funds from a checking account by writing a check or from a savings account by completing a slip and presenting a passbook is known as
a. deposit. c. withdrawal.
b. overdraft. d. credit.

_____ 44. A check that is so old when presented for payment that it is no longer valid is called a/an
a. postdated check. c. stale check.
b. old voucher. d. warrant.

_____ 45. A check that is not considered negotiable but can be converted into a negotiable instrument or cash is a/an
a. warrant. c. voucher.
b. note. d. limited check.

_____ 46. Withdrawal of funds from one account and transferring them to another, in specific amounts, at specified times, according to prior written agreement, is known as
a. automatic transfer of funds c. electronic funds transfer system.
b. bank by mail. d. point-of-sale banking.

_____ 47. A paperless computerized system enabling funds to be debited, credited, or transferred is known as
a. automatic transfer of funds. c. electronic funds transfer system.
b. bank by mail. d. automatic bill paying.

_____ 48. When an account holder has given the bank permission to transfer funds monthly for bill paying as a substitute for check writing, it is referred to as
   a. transfer payment system.
   b. pay-by-phone system.
   c. point-of-sale banking.
   d. automatic bill paying.

_____ 49. What is the name for a check which has been created from a digital image of the original?
   a. Counter check
   b. Certified check
   c. Money order
   d. Electronic check

_____ 50. On the back of a check or money order, the payee must write his name as it appears on the front. This is referred to as a/an
   a. deposit.
   b. endorsement.
   c. credit.
   d. debit.

_____ 51. What is the most common way of endorsing a check when the payee simply signs his name on the back?
   a. Full endorsement
   b. Restrictive endorsement
   c. Trailing endorsement
   d. Blank endorsement

_____ 52. What is the name for a special endorsement when a check (third-party check) is to be transferred to another person or company?
   a. Full endorsement
   b. Restrictive endorsement
   c. Trailing endorsement
   d. Blank endorsement

_____ 53. When a check is written and is not backed by funds in the bank, usually on new accounts, it is referred to as
   a. skipping.
   b. cheating.
   c. kiting.
   d. skimming.

_____ 54. When choosing a PIN for use with a bank account, be sure to
   a. use numbers that are found in your wallet.
   b. tell someone else in case you forget.
   c. include part of your social security number.
   d. none of the above.

_____ 55. When deposits are made, they are added to the balance of a bank account, or
   a. debited.
   b. credited.
   c. noted.
   d. drafted.

_____ 56. When checks are written or other withdrawals are made, they are subtracted from the bank balance, or
   a. debited.
   b. credited.
   c. noted.
   d. drafted.

_____ 57. You should call the patient and ask him to send a new check when you receive a/an
   a. limited check.
   b. cashier's check.
   c. disputed check.
   d. unsigned check.

_____ 58. On a monthly basis, to ensure accuracy of the bank balance, the bank statement should be
   a. taken to the bank.
   b. reconciled.
   c. brought to the attention of the physician.
   d. audited.

_____ 59. Amounts owed to creditors for the regular operation of a business are known as
   a. accounts receivable.
   b. accounts payable.
   c. capital.
   d. proprietorship.

60. Professional discounts, courtesy adjustments, and disallowances by insurance companies are examples of
a. liabilities.   c. adjustments.
b. credits.   d. assets.

61. In a manual bookkeeping system, copies of the ledger card can be used as
a. insurance bills.   c. day sheets.
b. patient statements.   d. receipts.

62. Accounting that is neither self-balancing nor well formulated is called
a. double-entry accounting.   c. accounts receivable.
b. single-entry accounting.   d. accounts payable.

63. Cash, inventory, furniture, and equipment are types of
a. assets.   c. vouchers.
b. collateral.   d. earnings.

64. Change for a patient who pays cash is made from the
a. petty cash fund.   c. deposit envelope.
b. bank.   d. change drawer.

65. For minor office expenses, money should be taken from the
a. bank.   c. petty cash fund.
b. checking account.   d. change drawer.

66. Recording the financial affairs of a business is the main purpose of all
a. medical record systems.   c. audits.
b. patient ledger cards.   d. bookkeeping systems.

67. Amounts paid out for the expenses of the medical practice are recorded in the
a. accounts receivable.   c. general ledger.
b. accounts payable ledger.   d. final ledger.

68. Payments at the time of service and payments received by mail must be recorded
a. daily.   c. monthly.
b. weekly.   d. yearly.

69. It is important that each day's cash and check receipts equals the day's total
a. payments.   c. assets.
b. bank deposit.   d. charges.

70. Each transaction to a daily ledger is recorded by the medical assistant or bookkeeper; this is also referred to as
a. crediting.   c. debiting.
b. archiving.   d. posting.

71. An unexpected, unplanned event that may involve injury is a/an
a. accident.   c. disability.
b. mishap.   d. illness.

72. Specific conditions listed in an insurance policy for which the policy will not pay are referred to as
a. exclusions.   c. extended benefits.
b. inclusions.   d. conversions.

73. What is the document called that the physician receives from private insurance carriers which details benefits that were paid or denied on an insurance claim?
a. Extended benefits   c. Explanation of benefits

b. Remittance advice   d. Summary notice

74. Payment made periodically to keep an insurance policy in force is referred to as the
   a. deductible.   c. contract payment.
   b. co-payment.   d. premium.

75. An illness or injury that prevents an insured person from performing all major duties of her occupation or from engaging in any other type of work for remuneration is known as
   a. partial disability.   c. preexisting condition.
   b. total disability.   d. temporary disability.

76. A clause in a group insurance policy that allows the insured to continue the same or lesser coverage under an individual policy is a/an
   a. preexisting clause.   c. reinstatement clause.
   b. conversion privilege.   d. group benefit.

77. An insurance policy is a legally enforceable
   a. attestment.   c. agreement or contract.
   b. consent or authorization.   d. condition.

78. An injury that occurred before the issuance of a health insurance policy is referred to as a/an
   a. preexisting benefit.   c. preexisting condition.
   b. permanent condition.   d. preexisting exclusion.

79. Claims may be received, edited, and distributed electronically to insurance companies through a central
   a. clearinghouse.   c. participating physician.
   b. insurance carrier.   d. physician network.

80. What is a method of payment for health services by which the health group is prepaid a contracted amount for each patient enrolled without consideration of the amount of service provided to each patient?
   a. Relative value study   c. Fee-for-service
   b. Usual, customary, and reasonable   d. Capitation

81. The process of finding out if a service or procedure is covered under a patient's insurance policy is
   a. predetermination.   c. preauthorization.
   b. precertification.   d. preexisting.

82. The process of finding out the maximum dollar amount that the insurance company will pay for the professional service to be rendered to the patient is called
   a. predetermination   c. preauthorization.
   b. precertification.   d. preexisting.

83. A voluntary prescription drug coverage plan falls under which part of the Medicare program?
   a. Part A   c. Part C
   b. Part B   d. Part D

84. Hospital insurance benefits to beneficiaries falls under which part of the Medicare program?
   a. Part A   c. Part C
   b. Part B   d. Part D

85. A health benefits program offering three types of plans for dependents of men and women in the military is called
   a. CHAMPVA.   c. TRICARE.
   b. Stark I.   d. Medigap.

_____ 86. A claim in which the patient is seen by the physician but may continue to work without limitations is a/an

    a. temporary disability claim.
    c. permanent disability claim.
    b. nondisability claim.
    d. stationary disability claim.

_____ 87. Health insurance claims can be submitted

    a. on paper.
    c. both a and b.
    b. electronically.
    d. neither a nor b.

_____ 88. A discussion with the patient and family concerning diagnosis, prognosis, risks, and/or instructions is referred to a/an

    a. consultation session.
    c. referral.
    b. counseling session.
    d. transfer of care.

_____ 89. The office manager

    a. has authority over the physician.
    b. oversees only the administrative staff.
    c. should use her position of authority to award her friends.
    d. acts as liaison between the employees and the physician.

_____ 90. Distractions may be minimized in an open-space office by

    a. facing desks away from high traffic areas.
    b. facing desks toward high traffic areas.
    c. lining desks up facing the reception area.
    d. none of the above.

_____ 91. How far ahead of an office meeting should the agenda be distributed to office employees for review?

    a. one week
    c. two or three days
    b. two or three hours
    d. two or three weeks

_____ 92. Generally, the minutes of an office meeting

    a. briefly outline the topics discussed at the meeting.
    b. state word-for-word what took place at the meeting.
    c. include notes containing the most important information.
    d. should not be typed until just prior to the next meeting.

_____ 93. Appropriate terminology and the basic format for taking minutes at an office meeting can be found in

    a. the _Physicians' Desk Reference_
    b. the American Secretaries Rules and Regulations
    c. _Robert's Rules of Order Newly Revised_
    d. the employee handbook

_____ 94. Copies of the minutes from an office meeting should be distributed to

    a. those who attended the meeting.
    c. all patients.
    b. only the physician.
    d. no one.

_____ 95. An employee handbook includes

    a. minutes of all staff meetings.
    b. personal hiring information on all employees.
    c. job descriptions.
    d. everything that the employees want the office manager to know about them.

_____ 96. An office procedures manual provides a compilation of

    a. job descriptions.
    c. the minutes from staff meetings.

b. sample forms for office tasks.   d. patient education brochures.

_____ 97. When storing office supplies, it is recommended to
a. use new packages of bond paper before the old packages.
b. stack boxes vertically.
c. position small items at eye level.
d. store everything in high humidity.

_____ 98. The medical staff is protected from on-the-job health and safety hazards by the rules set forth by the
a. Occupational Safety and Health Administration.
b. Occupational Health and Safety Administration.
c. Family and Medical Leave Act.
d. physician.

_____ 99. Airplane tickets purchased online can often be
a. totally nonrefundable.
b. refundable after 30 days.
c. exchanged for a different flight.
d. refundable with no penalty for up to a year.

_____ 100. It is important for the office manager to create a work atmosphere that is free of
a. discipline.   c. multicultural staff.
b. barriers and bias.   d. supervision.

_____ 101. What can help strengthen the office, attract new patients, and connect with a rapidly changing population?
a. Having staff that are all the same culture
b. An office manager who is over the age of 50
c. Multicultural staff
d. New physician

_____ 102. The Practice Information Brochure should
a. describe basic office policies.   c. act as a communication instrument.
b. avoid technical language.   d. all of the above.

_____ 103. A medical practice Web site should include information such as
a. patient education articles.   c. locations and contact information.
b. mission statement and services.   d. all of the above.

_____ 104. The seller of medical supplies will prepare a statement of item descriptions, amounts owed, quantity, price, and shipping date. This is called a/an
a. purchase order.   c. invoice.
b. order form.   d. packing list.

_____ 105. What is the control system called that includes an up-to-date list of all supplies, the number of items on the shelf, the reorder point, and the time required to fill an order?
a. Management control system   c. Supply control system
b. Invoice control system   d. Inventory control system

_____ 106. Quid pro quo, hostile environment, sexual favoritism, and harassment by nonemployees are all forms of
a. litigation.   c. sexual harassment.
b. confidentiality.   d. civil rights.

_____ 107. If the physician makes numerous trips out of town during the year, it may be very helpful to use the services of a local, reputable

	a. supply company.	c. accountant.
	b. travel agent.	d. hotel broker.

____108. Prepare for an interview of a job applicant by composing a standard
   a. list of open-ended questions.   c. policy handbook.
   b. training brochure.   d. list of job descriptions.

____109. Causes for dismissal or termination of an employee include
   a. willful disobedience.   c. business downturn.
   b. violation of company policies.   d. all of the above

____110. The law that sets Social Security taxes and benefits is the
   a. Family and Medical Leave Act.
   b. Federal Insurance Contributions Act (FICA).
   c. Americans with Disabilities Act.
   d. Federal Unemployment Tax Act.

____111. Legislation that provides for taxes to be collected at the federal level and which helps subsidize individual state's administration of their unemployment compensation programs is the
   a. Federal Withholding Tax.
   b. Federal Insurance Contributions Act (FICA).
   c. Federal Unemployment Tax Act (FUTA).
   d. Federal Labor Law.

____112. The tax deducted from an employee's gross income based on the number of withholding exemptions and amount earned for a pay period is called the
   a. Federal Withholding Tax.   c. Federal Tax Deposit Coupon.
   b. Federal Unemployment Tax.   d. Fair Labor Standards Act.

____113. The form identifying the employer, employee, gross earnings, and deductions for federal, state, FICA, and local income taxes is the
   a. Employee's Withholding Allowance Certificate.
   b. Wage and Tax Statement.
   c. Employer's Quarterly Federal Tax Return.
   d. Transmittal of Wage and Tax Statement.

____114. Each person in the United States is required to obtain a Social Security number
   a. at birth.   c. by the age of two.
   b. by the age of one.   d. by the age of five.

____115. The amount of Federal Unemployment Tax to be paid is stated in a federal publication entitled
   a. Wage and Tax Statement.
   b. Employer's Quarterly Federal Tax Return.
   c. Federal Tax Instructions.
   d. Employer's Tax Guide.

____116. A schedule of financial information required four times a year by the government is the
   a. Employers Quarterly Federal Tax Return.
   b. Transmittal of Wage and Tax Statement.
   c. Federal Income Tax.
   d. Profit and Loss Statement.

____117. The information given to employees at the end of an employment year, showing total wages and the amount of income tax withheld is called a/an
   a. Transmittal of Wage and Tax Statement (W-3).

b. Employee Withholding Allowance Certificate (W-4).

c. Wage and Tax Statement Form (W-2).

d. Employee's Earning Record.

_____118. Determining how long overdue accounts are is called
a. analyzing.
b. summarizing.
c. accounting.
d. aging.

_____119. A list of all account balances and the amounts owed to the medical practice is called a/an
a. accounts receivable report.
b. accounts payable report.
c. aging summary analysis.
d. insurance aging report.

_____120. To obtain a net income figure, subtract expenses from
a. yearly income.
b. gross income.
c. net income.
d. overhead expenses.

_____121. Wages, salaries, and benefits constitute a major portion of a practice's
a. income.
b. expenses.
c. capitation.
d. accounts receivable.

_____122. A nine-digit number used for federal tax accounting purposes is a/an
a. withholding number.
b. deduction number.
c. federal insurance contribution number.
d. employer identification number.

_____123. What is used to analyze practice productivity?
a. Collection ratio
b. Overhead expense ratio
c. Cost of procedures and services ratio
d. All of the above

_____124. One of the primary reasons that an employer will reject a job applicant includes
a. little interest or poor reasons for desiring a job.
b. professionalism.
c. good communication skills.
d. excellent spelling and legible handwriting.

_____125. How many employment opportunities in the United States are provided by health care and service-oriented medical fields?
a. 25%
b. 33%
c. 50%
d. 75%

_____126. How many job opportunities derive from personal contact (acquaintances)?
a. 65%
b. 75%
c. 85%
d. 95%

_____127. If an item on a job application does not apply or cannot be answered, the applicant should
a. make up an answer.
b. ask someone to clarify the question.
c. leave the item blank.
d. show the question has not been overlooked by inserting "no" or "NA."

_____128. When completing a job application form, the applicant should
a. fill the form out quickly to demonstrate how adept he is.
b. ignore the fine print.
c. read the entire application before beginning to fill it out.
d. skip sections that do not apply.

_____129. A letter of introduction should

a. list all explicit dates and facts about the applicant's work experience.
b. include salary expectations.
c. be brief and eye-catching.
d. none of the above

____130. A letter of introduction may be addressed to
a. the person most likely to be doing the interviewing.
b. Dear Office Manager.
c. Dear Members of the Personnel Committee.
d. any of the above.

____131. A cover letter should include
a. personal contact information.
b. height, weight, and gender.
c. information about the job applicant's family.
d. details of the job applicant's employment history.

____132. The resumé most familiar to employers and the easiest for the applicant to prepare is the
a. chronological resumé.
b. functional resumé.
c. combination resumé.
d. results-oriented resumé.

____133. Which resumé highlights qualifications and marketable skills but does not list specific job titles or descriptions with dates?
a. Chronological resumé
b. Functional resumé
c. Combination resumé
d. Results-oriented resumé

____134. Which resumé emphasizes both specific work experience and relevant medical skills?
a. Chronological resumé
b. Functional resumé
c. Combination resumé
d. Results-oriented resumé

____135. Which resumé focuses on accomplishments?
a. Chronological resumé
b. Functional resumé
c. Combination resumé
d. Results-oriented resumé

____136. A job application must be
a. neat.
b. accurate.
c. professional looking.
d. all of the above.

____137. Personal references should be people that
a. you know well.
b. can vouch for your character.
c. are able to speak truthfully.
d. all of the above.

____138. Which resumé is a hard-copy document designed to be scanned by an optical character reader and is then screened for specific keywords in order to pick applicants for personal interviews?
a. Electronic resumé
b. Scannable resumé
c. Functional resumé
d. Combination resumé

____139. An electronically formatted resumé can be easily sent by
a. telephone.
b. fax.
c. e-mail.
d. telegraph.

____140. The interview consists of several stages; the first stage is
a. establishing rapport.
b. greeting the interviewer.
c. learning all you can about the employer.
d. restating your interest.

_____141. If an interview question could be interpreted in more than one way, you should
    a. ask for clarification.   c. say that you just do not know.
    b. ask if you can come back to that one.   d. say the first thing that comes to mind.

_____142. Which of the following is an illegal question?
    a. Do you own a car?
    b. Are you considering having any more children?
    c. What church do you go to?
    d. All are illegal questions and do not have to be answered.

Matching

Match each term with the correct statement below.

a. dun
b. fee-for-service
c. fee schedule
d. garnishment
e. ledger card

f. multipurpose billing form
g. open accounts
h. quantum merit
i. receipt
j. skip

_____143. record for an individual account showing charges, payments, adjustments, and balances owed
_____144. debtor who has moved and left no forwarding address
_____145. attaching a debtor's property or wages for payment of a debt
_____146. combination bill, insurance form, and routing document
_____147. list of medical procedures and services and fees charged
_____148. written acknowledgment of payment
_____149. set amounts for each professional service

Match each term with the correct statement below.

a. electronic funds transfer system
b. forgery
c. limited check
d. overdraft
e. payee

f. payer
g. reconciliation
h. savings account
i. service charge
j. withdrawal

_____150. charge against an account in excess of the account balance
_____151. bank fee assessed for processing transactions and account maintenance
_____152. party responsible for payment of amount owed as shown on a check or note
_____153. person named on a draft or check as the recipient of the amount shown
_____154. act of proving the accuracy of the bank's records on an account by comparing bank figures with those of the customer, using mathematical adjustments
_____155. fraudulent signature or instrument
_____156. removal of funds
_____157. check that is void if written over a certain amount
_____158. interest-bearing account that does not offer check-writing capability
_____159. system by which preauthorized automatic transfers are made

Match each term with the correct statement below.

a. double-entry accounting
b. extend
c. general ledger
d. liability
e. open account
f. petty cash fund
g. post
h. proprietorship
i. single-entry accounting
j. voucher

____160. bookkeeping system of financial records used in business whereby equal debits and credits are recorded for each transaction

____161. to carry forward the balance of an individual ledger

____162. owner's net worth or equity; value of assets exceeding liability

____163. monies that are owed for business expenditures

____164. any account with a non-zero debit or credit balance

____165. to record or transfer financial entries, debit or credit, to an account

____166. form stating details as evidence of a disbursement of cash

____167. small cash fund readily available for minor office expenses

____168. easy bookkeeping system but not self-balancing nor well formulated

____169. journal in which all daily fees and payments may be recorded

Match each term with the correct statement below.

a. adjudicate
b. claim
c. coinsurance
d. co-payment
e. deductible
f. dependents
g. elimination period
h. exclusions
i. limitations
j. major medical

____170. to settle judicially as in a determination of payment in an insurance claim

____171. insurance policy especially designed to offset heavy medical expenses resulting from catastrophic or prolonged illness or injury

____172. type of cost sharing whereby the insured pays a specified amount per unit of service at the time services are rendered

____173. specific hazards, perils, or conditions listed in an insurance policy for which the company will not pay

____174. under an insurance contract, the spouse and children of the insured

____175. an amount the insured must pay in a calendar year before policy benefits begin

____176. request for payment under an insurance contract or bond

____177. cost-sharing requirement under a health insurance policy that stipulates the insured assume a percentage of the costs of covered services

Match each term with the correct statement below.

a. balance sheet
b. closed accounts
c. deduction
d. disbursement record
e. Employee Withholding Allowance Cert.
f. employer
g. employer identification number
h. exemption
i. Federal Insurance Contributions Act
j. Federal Unemployment Tax Act

_____178. chronological register of monthly business expenditures and yearly totals
_____179. one who hires people to work for wages or a salary
_____180. amount withheld from an employee's gross income for income tax purposes
_____181. presents the financial position of the medical practice
_____182. deduction from gross income allowed a taxpayer that reduces the amount of income on which the individual is taxed
_____183. tax that pays to run state unemployment programs; deposits made quarterly
_____184. form W-4; states number of exemptions claimed
_____185. payroll tax which finances elderly and retirement benefits
_____186. accounts with zero balances
_____187. nine-digit number used for tax accounting purposes

Match each term with the correct statement below.

a. blind letter
b. chronological resumé
c. cover letter
d. diplomate
e. electronic job search
f. employee handbook
g. employment agency
h. format
i. functional resumé
j. human resources department
k. performance evaluation
l. portfolio
m. results-oriented resumé
n. resumé

_____188. personnel office
_____189. lists expectations for job performances; sets guidelines for salary increases; and sets standards for equal employment opportunity, affirmative action, and minority employment
_____190. periodic summary of an employee's work habits and behaviors
_____191. compilation of items that represents a job applicant's skills
_____192. summary of education, skills, and work experience, usually in outline form
_____193. shape, size, and makeup of a letter, report, or document
_____194. physician certified in a field of specialization by a medical board
_____195. in job seeking, a letter of introduction prepared to accompany a resumé
_____196. computerized service for obtaining job listings and career advice
_____197. business organization that refers job applicants to potential employers
_____198. communication expressing an interest in a job should one become available
_____199. job seeking data sheet that focuses on accomplishments
_____200. job seeking data sheet that focuses on skills, not job titles

Completion
Complete each statement.

201. Obtain a complete and accurate _____ _____ from the patient at the time of the first visit, securing enough personal and financial history to be able to trace a patient who moves.

202. _____ _____ are companies that keep records on individual borrowers.

203. If unable to trace and contact a patient, turn the patient's financial information over to a/an _____ _____ immediately.

204. _____ _____ is a principle that means "as much as he deserves."

205. In most situations, insurers and the government ban waiving the _____ amount.

206. The office should have a/an _____ in order to accurately prepare bank deposits, post charges and payments, or add totals on an order form.

207. A/an _____ _____ is a business that pursues payment on delinquent accounts when the physician's office has come to a dead end in the collection process.

208. A medical practice may decide to file a claim in _____ _____ court rather than turn it over to a collection agency.

209. _____ laws are federal laws, and a patient who is unable to pay debts and files becomes a ward of the federal court and is protected by the court.

210. A/An _____ _____ is a check for use in traveling when personal checks may not be accepted and carrying large amounts of cash is not desirable.

211. _____ is a system that is a substitute for check writing whereby the medical assistant telephones the bank or savings and loan association to make payments.

212. When preparing a/an _____, verify that the back of each check or money order has been endorsed properly.

213. A/An _____ _____ service is the automatic deposit of wages or benefits into a customer's bank account.

214. ATM _____ occurs when thieves use portable card-reading devices that fit over the card slot to record data on a card's magnetic strip.

215. When each check is written, be sure to complete the _____ or stub attached to the check for proper record keeping.

216. Banking _____ gives the user access via the Internet to some banking services 24 hours a day, 7 days a week.

217. Every month, a/an _____ _____ is received which lists the date and amount of each deposit and each withdrawal.

218. The main purpose of any _____ system is to record the financial affairs of the business.

219. Places of business that offer merchandise for sale keep accounts on a/an _____ _____, which means that income is considered earned when the merchandise is sold.

220. Physicians' accounts are kept on what is called a/an _____ _____, to indicate what happens to the money taken in.

221. Traditional _____ insurance is protection against injury or loss of health.

222. The oldest and most popular of all the prepaid health plans are _____ _____ _____.

223. The _____ _____ is the time frame after the beginning date of a policy before benefits for illness or injury become payable.

224. The _____ program is designed for needy and low-income people, the blind, the disabled, and families receiving aid to dependent children.

225. The _____ for a staff meeting should be prepared with input from all staff members to speed discussion and diffuse office conflicts.

226. Most employers require a 60- to 90-day _____ period to determine whether a new employee is able to perform all job duties satisfactorily.

227. Regularly scheduled _____ _____ are important in establishing a pattern of positive interaction among staff members.

228. A/An _____ _____ _____ is a blueprint for evacuating the premises and recovery of valuable documents should a catastrophe strike.

229. A/An _____ _____ is a written authorization to a merchant to deliver merchandise, materials, or services at an agreed-upon price.

230. Any conduct in the workplace that occurs because of a person's _____ is sexual discrimination and is prohibited by Title VII of the Civil Rights Act of 1964.

231. Some physicians prefer that a medical assistant use a manual _____ check writing and payroll journal system. This is a type of pegboard bookkeeping system which combines check writing with an itemized account of all deductions.

232. Some physicians provide _____ benefits for their employees, consisting of partial or full payment of health insurance, life insurance, and so on.

233. It is important to have a/an _____ for the medical office which is devised from analyzing last year's expenses and income and then projecting the needs of the practice for the upcoming year.

234. The office manager needs to keep a close eye on the balance of the _____ to make sure enough money is on hand for payment of payroll, overhead, and other office expenses.

235. The _____ job market is the network or grapevine of contacts through which hiring is often done.

236. To post a resumé _____, upload the resumé using a file-transfer feature of the software, following the computer manual directions.

237. A job seeker can visit the _____ _____ Department of local medical facilities to check job postings on personnel bulletin boards.

238. The two best options for electronic resumés are the _____ and the _____ versions.

239. The purpose of a/an _____ is to provide additional documentation in support of information provided in the resumé. It often includes evidence of skills such as projects done in a classroom, tests, completed insurance claims and so forth.

240. Letters of _____ from previous employers are an excellent item to keep in a portfolio and should be updated frequently.

Short Answer

241. List the four basic steps to file a claim in small claims court.

242. List the four options the patient has after being served by small claims court.

243. Name two ways that the Federal Wage Garnishment Law protects the debtor.

244. Name five types of inaccurate accounting entries (errors) that might be found to help solve a posting error.

245. Describe the steps used to establish an accounts receivable control to verify posting and balances.

246. List the seven items that must be contained in an itemized statement.

247. The six variables used for DRG (diagnosis related group) classifications are:

248. Describe one of the three programs financed from one payroll tax (FICA) to which employers and employees contribute at a rate specified by law.

249. List five job performance areas that are included when an employer evaluates a new employee's work performance at the end of the 90-day probation period.

250. Name one suggestion for handling an illegal question if it were to be asked by an interviewer.

Exam 4
Answer Section

TRUE/FALSE

1.	ANS: F	PTS:	1
2.	ANS: T	PTS:	1
3.	ANS: F	PTS:	1
4.	ANS: T	PTS:	1
5.	ANS: T	PTS:	1
6.	ANS: F	PTS:	1
7.	ANS: T	PTS:	1
8.	ANS: T	PTS:	1
9.	ANS: F	PTS:	1
10.	ANS: F	PTS:	1
11.	ANS: F	PTS:	1
12.	ANS: T	PTS:	1

13. ANS: F   PTS: 1
14. ANS: F   PTS: 1
15. ANS: T   PTS: 1
16. ANS: F   PTS: 1
17. ANS: T   PTS: 1
18. ANS: T   PTS: 1
19. ANS: T   PTS: 1
20. ANS: F   PTS: 1

MULTIPLE CHOICE

21. ANS: A   PTS: 1
22. ANS: C   PTS: 1
23. ANS: B   PTS: 1
24. ANS: C   PTS: 1
25. ANS: A   PTS: 1
26. ANS: B   PTS: 1
27. ANS: C   PTS: 1
28. ANS: B   PTS: 1
29. ANS: C   PTS: 1
30. ANS: D   PTS: 1
31. ANS: B   PTS: 1
32. ANS: C   PTS: 1
33. ANS: A   PTS: 1
34. ANS: B   PTS: 1
35. ANS: D   PTS: 1
36. ANS: D   PTS: 1
37. ANS: B   PTS: 1
38. ANS: A   PTS: 1
39. ANS: C   PTS: 1
40. ANS: A   PTS: 1
41. ANS: B   PTS: 1
42. ANS: A   PTS: 1
43. ANS: C   PTS: 1
44. ANS: C   PTS: 1
45. ANS: A   PTS: 1
46. ANS: A   PTS: 1
47. ANS: C   PTS: 1
48. ANS: D   PTS: 1
49. ANS: A   PTS: 1
50. ANS: B   PTS: 1
51. ANS: D   PTS: 1
52. ANS: A   PTS: 1

53. ANS: C   PTS: 1
54. ANS: D   PTS: 1
55. ANS: B   PTS: 1
56. ANS: A   PTS: 1
57. ANS: D   PTS: 1
58. ANS: B   PTS: 1
59. ANS: B   PTS: 1
60. ANS: C   PTS: 1
61. ANS: B   PTS: 1
62. ANS: B   PTS: 1
63. ANS: A   PTS: 1
64. ANS: D   PTS: 1
65. ANS: C   PTS: 1
66. ANS: D   PTS: 1
67. ANS: B   PTS: 1
68. ANS: A   PTS: 1
69. ANS: B   PTS: 1
70. ANS: D   PTS: 1
71. ANS: A   PTS: 1
72. ANS: A   PTS: 1
73. ANS: C   PTS: 1
74. ANS: D   PTS: 1
75. ANS: B   PTS: 1
76. ANS: B   PTS: 1
77. ANS: C   PTS: 1
78. ANS: C   PTS: 1
79. ANS: A   PTS: 1
80. ANS: D   PTS: 1
81. ANS: B   PTS: 1
82. ANS: A   PTS: 1
83. ANS: D   PTS: 1
84. ANS: A   PTS: 1
85. ANS: C   PTS: 1
86. ANS: B   PTS: 1
87. ANS: C   PTS: 1
88. ANS: B   PTS: 1
89. ANS: D   PTS: 1
90. ANS: A   PTS: 1
91. ANS: C   PTS: 1
92. ANS: C   PTS: 1
93. ANS: C   PTS: 1
94. ANS: A   PTS: 1
95. ANS: C   PTS: 1

96.	ANS: B	PTS: 1
97.	ANS: C	PTS: 1
98.	ANS: A	PTS: 1
99.	ANS: A	PTS: 1
100.	ANS: B	PTS: 1
101.	ANS: C	PTS: 1
102.	ANS: D	PTS: 1
103.	ANS: D	PTS: 1
104.	ANS: C	PTS: 1
105.	ANS: D	PTS: 1
106.	ANS: C	PTS: 1
107.	ANS: B	PTS: 1
108.	ANS: A	PTS: 1
109.	ANS: D	PTS: 1
110.	ANS: B	PTS: 1
111.	ANS: C	PTS: 1
112.	ANS: A	PTS: 1
113.	ANS: B	PTS: 1
114.	ANS: C	PTS: 1
115.	ANS: D	PTS: 1
116.	ANS: A	PTS: 1
117.	ANS: C	PTS: 1
118.	ANS: D	PTS: 1
119.	ANS: A	PTS: 1
120.	ANS: B	PTS: 1
121.	ANS: B	PTS: 1
122.	ANS: D	PTS: 1
123.	ANS: D	PTS: 1
124.	ANS: A	PTS: 1
125.	ANS: C	PTS: 1
126.	ANS: B	PTS: 1
127.	ANS: D	PTS: 1
128.	ANS: C	PTS: 1
129.	ANS: C	PTS: 1
130.	ANS: D	PTS: 1
131.	ANS: A	PTS: 1
132.	ANS: A	PTS: 1
133.	ANS: B	PTS: 1
134.	ANS: C	PTS: 1
135.	ANS: D	PTS: 1
136.	ANS: D	PTS: 1
137.	ANS: D	PTS: 1
138.	ANS: B	PTS: 1

139. ANS: C   PTS: 1
140. ANS: B   PTS: 1
141. ANS: A   PTS: 1
142. ANS: D   PTS: 1

MATCHING

143. ANS: E   PTS: 1
144. ANS: J   PTS: 1
145. ANS: D   PTS: 1
146. ANS: F   PTS: 1
147. ANS: C   PTS: 1
148. ANS: I   PTS: 1
149. ANS: B   PTS: 1

150. ANS: D   PTS: 1
151. ANS: I   PTS: 1
152. ANS: F   PTS: 1
153. ANS: E   PTS: 1
154. ANS: G   PTS: 1
155. ANS: B   PTS: 1
156. ANS: J   PTS: 1
157. ANS: C   PTS: 1
158. ANS: H   PTS: 1
159. ANS: A   PTS: 1

160. ANS: A   PTS: 1
161. ANS: B   PTS: 1
162. ANS: H   PTS: 1
163. ANS: D   PTS: 1
164. ANS: E   PTS: 1
165. ANS: G   PTS: 1
166. ANS: J   PTS: 1
167. ANS: F   PTS: 1
168. ANS: I   PTS: 1
169. ANS: C   PTS: 1

170. ANS: A   PTS: 1
171. ANS: J   PTS: 1
172. ANS: D   PTS: 1
173. ANS: H   PTS: 1
174. ANS: F   PTS: 1
175. ANS: E   PTS: 1

176.	ANS: B	PTS: 1
177.	ANS: C	PTS: 1
178.	ANS: D	PTS: 1
179.	ANS: F	PTS: 1
180.	ANS: C	PTS: 1
181.	ANS: A	PTS: 1
182.	ANS: H	PTS: 1
183.	ANS: J	PTS: 1
184.	ANS: E	PTS: 1
185.	ANS: I	PTS: 1
186.	ANS: B	PTS: 1
187.	ANS: G	PTS: 1
188.	ANS: J	PTS: 1
189.	ANS: F	PTS: 1
190.	ANS: K	PTS: 1
191.	ANS: L	PTS: 1
192.	ANS: N	PTS: 1
193.	ANS: H	PTS: 1
194.	ANS: D	PTS: 1
195.	ANS: C	PTS: 1
196.	ANS: E	PTS: 1
197.	ANS: G	PTS: 1
198.	ANS: A	PTS: 1
199.	ANS: M	PTS: 1
200.	ANS: I	PTS: 1

COMPLETION

201. ANS: registration form

PTS: 1

202. ANS: Credit bureaus

PTS: 1

203. ANS: collection agency

PTS: 1

204. ANS: Quantum merit

PTS: 1

205. ANS: co-payment

PTS: 1

206. ANS: calculator

PTS: 1

207. ANS: collection agency

PTS: 1

208. ANS: small claims

PTS: 1

209. ANS: Bankruptcy

PTS: 1

210. ANS: traveler's check

PTS: 1

211. ANS: Pay-by-phone

PTS: 1

212. ANS:
deposit
bank deposit

PTS: 1

213. ANS: direct deposit

PTS: 1

214. ANS: skimming

PTS: 1

215. ANS: voucher

PTS: 1

216. ANS: online

PTS: 1

217. ANS: bank statement

PTS: 1

218. ANS: bookkeeping

PTS: 1

219. ANS: accrual basis

PTS: 1

220. ANS: cash basis

   PTS: 1
221. ANS: indemnity

   PTS: 1
222. ANS:
   health maintenance organizations
   HMOs

   PTS: 1
223. ANS: waiting period

   PTS: 1
224. ANS: Medicaid

   PTS: 1
225. ANS: agenda

   PTS: 1
226. ANS: probationary

   PTS: 1
227. ANS: staff meetings

   PTS: 1
228. ANS: disaster response plan

   PTS: 1
229. ANS: purchase order

   PTS: 1
230. ANS:
   gender
   sex

   PTS: 1
231. ANS: write-it-once

   PTS: 1
232. ANS: fringe

   PTS: 1
233. ANS: budget

PTS: 1
234. ANS: checkbook

PTS: 1
235. ANS: hidden

PTS: 1
236. ANS: online

PTS: 1
237. ANS: Human Resources

PTS: 1
238. ANS: ASCII, HTML

PTS: 1
239. ANS: portfolio

PTS: 1
240. ANS: recommendation

PTS: 1

SHORT ANSWER

241. ANS:
(a) Obtain a form from the clerk's office located at the Municipal or Justice Court. (b) File the initiating papers. (c) Pay the filing fee. (d) Make arrangements to serve the defendant.

PTS: 1
242. ANS:
(a) Pay the claim to the court clerk. (b) Ignore the claim and the physician will win by default.
(c) Request a small claims hearing and the court clerk will let both parties know when to appear.
(d) Demand a jury trial.

PTS: 1
243. ANS:
a) Limits the amount of earnings that can be garnished per pay period.
b) Protects the employee from being dismissed by the employer.

PTS: 1
244. ANS:
Any five accounting entries from the following list:
(a) figure that was missed
(b) miskeyed figure

(c) transposition in figures

(d) amount divisible by 9 that may indicate a transposed number

(e) figures in wrong columns

(f) amount divisible by 2 that may indicate posting in the wrong column

(g) sliding number (e.g., 500 instead of 50).

PTS: 1

245. ANS:

(a) Total the balances of all patient account records (ledgers) that indicate a balance due.

(b) Compare that total with the ending total of the accounts receivable figure on the daysheet; the two totals should agree.

(c) If the two totals are not in agreement, recheck the arithmetic on all ledger cards.

PTS: 1

246. ANS:

a) Provider's name

b) Date of services

c) Description of services and/or supplies with appropriate code numbers

d) Fee for each service or supply item

e) Diagnosis for which treatment is being received with appropriate code numbers

f) Number or frequency of each service

g) Place of treatment

PTS: 1

247. ANS:

a) Patient's principal diagnosis

b) Patient's secondary diagnosis

c) Surgical procedures

d) Comorbidity and complications

e) Age and sex

f) Discharge status

PTS: 1

248. ANS:

Any one of the following:

(a) Old Age Survivors and Disabilities Insurance (OASDI) provides the elderly with retirement benefits and their surviving dependents with survivors' benefits. (b) Hospital Insurance (HI) or Medicare program provides hospitalization insurance for the elderly. (c) The public Disability Insurance (DI) program provides workers with insurance if they become disabled during their working years.

PTS: 1

249. ANS:

Any five of the following:

(a) attendance and punctuality

(b) quality and quantity of work

(c) ability to work as a team member
(d) attitude toward coworkers and patients
(e) technical knowledge
(f) written and oral expression
(g) appearance

PTS: 1

250. ANS:
Any of the following:
(a) Answer the question, ignoring the fact that you know it is illegal.
(b) State that you think the question has no relevance to the requirements of the position.
(c) Refuse to answer and consider contacting an Equal Employment Opportunity office.

PTS: 1

CPSIA information can be obtained
at www.ICGtesting.com
Printed in the USA
LVHW071510261222
735880LV00016B/54

9 781497 433885